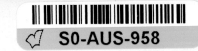

THE MOST DYNAMIC AND EFFECTIVE
NEW EXERCISE REGIMEN TODAY!

As star athletes can testify, exercise *doesn't* have to hurt to do your body good—not when you waterpower your workout! And you don't have to be a swimmer to reap the benefits of nature's nautilus machine. Water's gentle resistance supercharges *any* body movements; its buoyancy allows you to run, jump, bounce, and stretch your way to fitness without stressing delicate joints. Best of all, water's natural undulation provides exercising muscles with a constant hydro-massage, so you shape up, trim down, and develop aerobic fitness virtually painlessly. So take the plunge—for aerobics, sports training, pregnancy exercise, pain relief, or weight loss.

THE
WATERPOWER
WORKOUT

LYNDA HUEY is the athletic director of the International Sports Medicine Institute in Los Angeles, and is head of the AquaAerobic Program. She has co-hosted "Alive and Well" on the USA Network and was liaison between athletes and foreign delegations in the 1984 Olympics.

R. R. KNUDSON has written several young adult novels and is the co-author of several popular fitness guides.

THE WATERPOWER WORKOUT

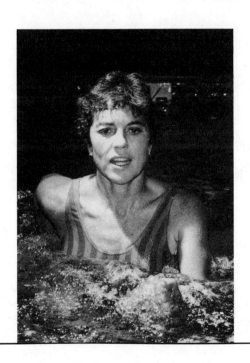

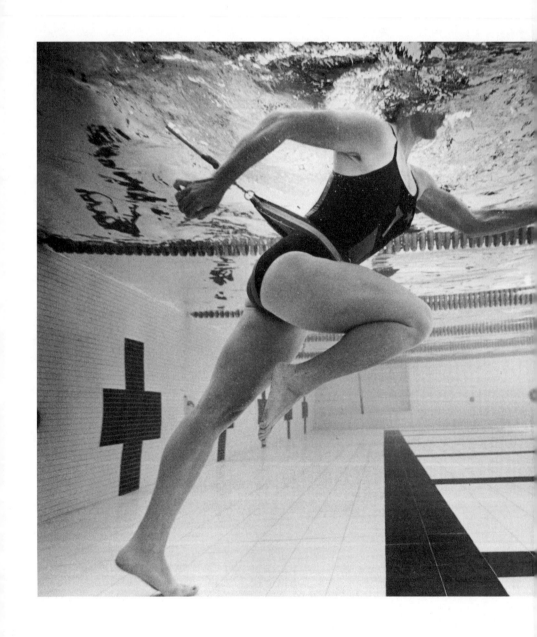

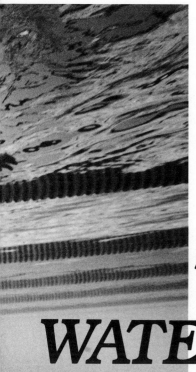

Lynda Huey
with R. R. Knudson

FOREWORD BY LEROY R. PERRY, JR., D.C.

PHOTOGRAPHS BY GLENN S. CAPERS

THE
WATERPOWER
WORKOUT

A PLUME BOOK

NEW AMERICAN LIBRARY

NEW YORK AND SCARBOROUGH, ONTARIO

PLUME TRADEMARK REG. U.S. PAT. OFF. AND FOREIGN COUNTRIES
REG. TRADEMARK—MARCA REGISTRADA
HECHO EN HARRISONBURG, VA., U.S.A.

SIGNET, SIGNET CLASSIC, MENTOR, PLUME, MERIDIAN and NAL BOOKS
are published *in the United States* by New American Library,
1633 Broadway, New York, New York 10019, *in Canada* by
The New American Library of Canada Limited,
81 Mack Avenue, Scarborough, Ontario M1L 1M8

Library of Congress Cataloging-in-Publication Data

Huey, Linda.
    The waterpower workout.

    I. Aquatic exercises.   2. Aerobic exercises.
I. Knudson, R. Rozanne, 1932–   . II. Title.
RA781.17.H84   1986   613.7'1   86-2360
ISBN 0-452-25828-6

Designed by Barbara Huntley

First Printing, June, 1986
    2   3   4   5   6   7   8   9
PRINTED IN THE UNITED STATES OF AMERICA

For my mentors:
    Bud, Tommie, Allan, Wiltie,
Ron, Zan, and RoMa

ACKNOWLEDGMENTS

Craig Nelson, Ph.D. and David Luna, *for their contributions to the original water exercise program.*

Doreen Rivera, *for suggestions on prenatal exercise.*

Pat Connolly, *for her coaching and training knowledge.*

RoMa Johnson *for assistance with the manuscript and her irrepressible good cheer.*

Mom, *who taught me years ago that if all else fails, "Go soak your head."*

International Sportsmedicine Institute; University of California, Irvine; Electro-Medical, Inc./18433 Amistad/Fountain Valley, CA *for pools, Acuscopes, and Myopulses.*

Arena, Zeta Zukki, and Bare Assets *for bathing suits and swim accessories.*

CONTENTS

FOREWORD by Leroy R. Perry, Jr., D.C.   xiii

1. WATER MAGIC   1

2. SHOWER EXERCISES   21

3. WATER STRETCH   27

4. THE BASIC WATERPOWER WORKOUT   41

5. WATER AEROBICS   69

6. EIGHT TIPS FOR IMPROVED WATERPOWER   83

7. SPORT-SPECIFIC WATER TRAINING   93

8. WATER REHABILITATION   115

9. ARTHRITIS WATER THERAPY   137

10. PRENATAL WATERPOWER   145

11. THE HOT TUB WORKOUT   169

POSTSCRIPT: THE JOY OF WATERPOWER   183

INDEX   185

FOREWORD

When Lynda Huey became athletic director at my International Sportsmedicine Institute in West Los Angeles, we shared our water training experience with professional and Olympic athletes, and with my patients. Almost everyone who came to the Institute was urged to use water as part of a training or rehabilitation program. We showed runners, cyclists, triathletes, tennis players, golfers, gymnasts, football players, hurdlers, and pole vaulters how to use water as their safety valve: They could take a day off without really taking a day off. They could avoid the normal stress and trauma of their sports while maintaining cardiovascular and muscular fitness in the water one day or more a week. Patients, particularly back-pain patients, used the Perry-Band, Perry Flotation Belt, face mask, and snorkel to swim in a posture-controlled position that helped them strengthen their abdominals, inner thighs, arms, and legs. This strength brought muscular balance to my patients' bodies, helping to eliminate back pain and other problems.

As demand grew for organized water-training sessions, Lynda and I developed a series of classes in the Institute's pools. Day by day these Aqua Aerobics classes grew, drawing participants from various fitness backgrounds. Some of these new members of our classes were just beginning a fitness program after years—or even lifetimes—of inactivity. Some were overweight and seeking ways to lose body fat. Others were pregnant or returning to shape after pregnancy. Businessmen and women, high school students who played intramural sports as well as post-surgical patients attended our classes, mingling with gold medalists and professional baseball and football players from all over the country. We found that water was a great equalizer. All these people with varied fitness levels could stretch and exercise together, each person working to his or her own level against water's resistance.

Eventually Lynda set down on paper her basic Waterpower Workout, later modifying it to develop programs for the injured, overweight, and pregnant, and suggesting extra aerobic work for athletes and others who asked for it. These modifications can be found in the chapters on Water Stretch, Prenatal Waterpower, Water Aerobics, and Sport-Specific Exercises.

Her excellent Waterpower has thus become a part of the lives of an increasing number of people—fitness "rookies" to world-class athletes. Some of those with whom Lynda and I have worked are pictured in the chapters to follow.

Evelyn Ashford—1984 Olympic gold medalist, 100 meters, 400 meter Relay.

Bernie Casey—Wide Receiver, San Francisco 49ers and Los Angeles Rams. Actor, co-starred in *Sharkey's Machine* and *Never Say Never Again.*

Wilt Chamberlain—the greatest basketball player of all time.

Bart Gallagher—Kim Gallagher's brother and coach. Now a writer, model, and actor.

Kim Gallagher—1984 Olympic silver medalist, 800 meters.

Marlene Harmon—1980 Olympic pentathlete.

Alberto Juantorena—1976 gold medalist for Cuba, 400 meters, 800 meters.

Murray Rose—1956, 1960 gold medalist for Australia, swimming. Voted Greatest Australian Male Olympian of All Time in 1983.

Mac Wilkins—1976 Olympic gold medalist, discus; 1984 Olympic silver medalist, discus.

Ruth Wysocki—1984 Olympian, 800 meters, 1500 meters.

Dr. Mike Greenberg—1984 Olympic team doctor; founder of the Clinic for Fitness Education; private practice in Brentwood, California.

Dr. Vicky Vodon—1984 Olympic team doctor; former UCLA athletic trainer; private practices in Los Angeles and Huntington Beach, California.

I believe that water exercise and Perry-Band/Perry Flotation Belt swimming have saved many patients from surgery and countless athletes from potential injuries. Now you, too, can do Lynda Huey's The *Waterpower Workout* in your own pool, hot tub, or even bathtub. Regular use of Waterpower programs will make you healthier, fitter, and a better athlete. *The Waterpower Workout* will change your life.

Leroy R. Perry, Jr., D.C.
Los Angeles, California

THE WATERPOWER WORKOUT

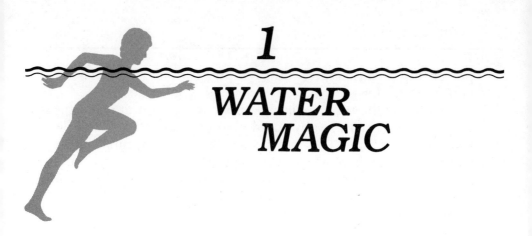

1
WATER MAGIC

September 1974: Carlsbad, California

Patty Van Wolvelaere, my teammate on Wilt Chamberlain's WonderWomen Track Club, was America's best hurdler. It was a joy working out with her, learning new training methods. We lived on the beach, so it was natural to do some of our workouts there.

Top sprinter Steve Williams was a transplanted New Yorker who was discovering beach workouts with us. One day we took him for a barefoot run down our wide, flat beach. As a wave rolled in, we lifted our knees and sprinted over the foam. As the wave receded, we jogged. We played with the waves like that for several miles, doing sprint drills as each wave broke. Then we walked back up the beach in knee-deep water, enjoying the sight of the sun on our shining thighs as they forcefully contracted, pulling us through the water.

Water adds magic to any workout. The magic lies in water's **resistance** to bodily movements, water's **support** for the body, and water's wonderful **freshness**. Submerged in water, you can quickly sense water's magic.

Water's buoyancy supports you as you move through it in a training program. Water's buoyancy lets you run, walk, jump, bounce, stretch, pivot—make any movement—without the jolts that could cause injuries if they were to occur on land. Water acts as a cushion for your weight-bearing joints, preventing strain, injury, and reinjury common to other exercise programs.

At the same time water is supporting you, it is resisting you. Any movement at any speed in any direction is slowed by water's resistance. This resistance causes your muscles to work harder than if you were simply moving your arms and legs through air. As you demand more from your muscles they adapt to the demand by becoming stronger. In addition to strengthening your body, you are burning calories, more calories than if you did exercises without resistance. Water is, in effect, a natural Universal Gym. Or a natural Nautilus machine that is instantly variable, depending on how much resistance (weight) you want to work against: the harder you push and pull and sweep and kick in the water, the more resistance you will meet from the water.

On land, such resistance would raise your body's temperature; and raise it further as you worked harder and longer during a training session. But with water's freshness, your body remains cool and soothed as if by massage.

With Waterpower, you'll experience water's magic right away. There are no preliminary weeks of exercising—no bending, stretching, slow walks or jogs you must do to get into shape before you enter the water. **You don't even have to be able to swim.**

TEST WATER'S POWER

To test the power of water, try this at home.

1. Draw a bucketful of warm water the next time you're watching TV. Rotate your ankles smoothly clockwise in the water. Rotate your ankles counterclockwise. Squeeze your toes together and curl them downward. Reach up with your toes and try to separate them as much as possible. Next, plunge one of your hands into the bucket, make a fist, then stretch your fingers as wide as possible. Repeat these stretches and contractions slowly 10 times,

rest for a minute, then repeat. (Or, fill the bucket with ice water and exercise a wrist or ankle that you may have strained slightly.)

2. Move to the bathroom and draw a tubful of water. Use it as a pool for stretching your arms, legs, and back. Stretch them as you have probably already learned to stretch before and after a weight workout or a run. Add more hot water, slide down to cover your body to your chin, and use your own tub as a hot tub. Stretch your shoulders and neck and allow the warm water to relax them. Give yourself a foot and hand massage. Breathe deeply.

3. Stand a minute, evaluating the effects. Surely your body feels relaxed and energized—fresher than before.

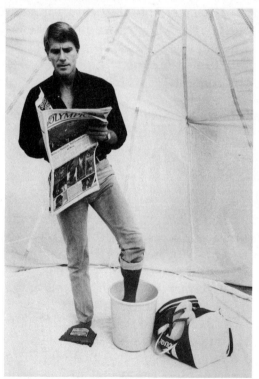

Waterpower refreshes Murray Rose's tired feet.

Multiply these sensations by the 10 to 45 minutes it takes to complete a water workout in a pool where you'll be able to work *every* muscle. After a single workout you will feel more flexible, agile, and powerful. These rewards and many others will make you look and feel better each day of your life.

WATERPOWER IS WHAT YOU NEED

As you turn the pages of *The Waterpower Workout*, you will see people doing 91 water exercises that are building their strength and power, controlling their weight, increasing their cardiovascular endurance, improving their flexibility, agility, balance, and coordination, or healing their injuries.

Consider the relaxed and joyful facial expressions of the people in water, their healthy, fit, beautiful bodies. These are not models, but terrific athletes who exercise often in water, who use it for general conditioning and for rehabilitating their injuries sustained on land. Notice the variety and number of exercises they do in water, the variety of their water gyms.

Soon you, too, will be using water's resistance, buoyancy, and freshness to achieve your own fitness goals.

CHOOSE YOUR PROGRAM

Now that you've decided Waterpower is for you, it's time to identify the specific program that will meet your immediate fitness or rehabilitation goals. You may have clearly specialized concerns—those of a competitive or injured athlete, a pregnant woman, or a person with arthritis. You may be looking for a completely new approach to weight control and fitness. You may be a recreational athlete who wants to add the power of water to your varied training schedule.

Whatever your needs, *The Waterpower Workout* has something to offer you. I've developed eight different Waterpower programs tailored to special fitness requirements. It should be easy to determine which program is right for you:

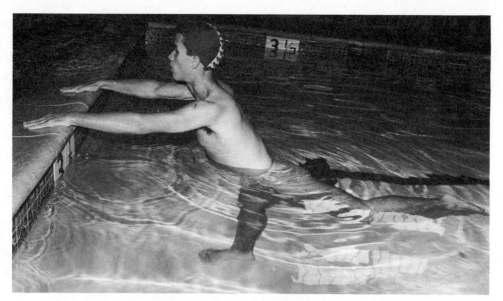

If you're afraid of water, begin by holding the side of the pool.

WATER STRETCH You should start with this program if you haven't exercised in many years, if you are overweight, afraid of water, or hesitant to begin a fitness program that jars the body. Water Stretch is gentle enough for post-surgical or other convalescent therapy. The gentle movements of Water Stretch will increase your strength, balance, and flexibility, and prepare you for a more rigorous and challenging workout. Once you're in condition, you can progress to the Basic Water Workout and use Water Stretch to warm up and warm down.

THE BASIC WATER WORKOUT If you're generally in shape, if you train regularly, or even if you are a highly conditioned athlete, use this multipurpose, well-rounded program. It can be modified for your individual needs simply by increasing or decreasing the number of repetitions of each exercise. Additionally, you can put more or less effort into each workout simply by deciding to work more or less powerfully against the water's resistance.

If you are a recreational athlete who has been, say, playing tennis or racquetball faithfully four times a week for many years, and you want to boost your enthusiasm and stamina, substitute the Basic Water Workout for one or more of your tennis or racquetball matches each week.

You may be a serious cyclist, triathlete, runner, cross-country skier, or other athlete training for a specific event. Perhaps you've nearly reached the upper limit of your capacity to handle your difficult workouts. If you add much more workload, you're likely to become injured. Nevertheless, **you want more.** Use the Basic Water Workout as a supplemental conditioning program once or twice a week to intensify training without incurring the risks.

WATER AEROBICS If you strengthen your muscles with weight training or other exercise and specifically seek aerobic conditioning from your water workout, use the Water Aerobics program. It offers you a 20-minute plan that will focus your efforts on strengthening your heart and lungs. Although the Basic Water Workout includes a substantial aerobic component, it also provides exercises for all major muscle groups of the body and takes 45 minutes or more for completion. If you're short on time, you'll get the most specific cardiovascular benefit from Water Aerobics.

If inclement weather forces you inside, find an indoor pool and substitute Water Aerobics for your usual sports until the weather warms up again.

SPORT-SPECIFIC WATER TRAINING Water Exercises can aid in strengthening your body and improving your technique in any specific sport. Used in conjunction with the Basic Water Workout and Water Aerobics, these exercises will improve your performance in many sports, from basketball to golf.

WATER REHABILITATION Follow the guidelines to this program if you're an athlete with an injury that prevents you from

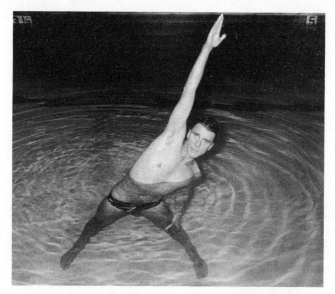

*Waterpower helps everyone from post-surgery
patients to Olympic athletes.*

training in your sport and you want to maintain your muscle
strength and cardiovascular fitness while you let your injury
heal. Begin by doing an exercise that will help your injured
body part become stronger, then add the Basic Water Workout
and Water Aerobics as a powerful substitute for your land-
sport training.

Water Rehabilitation can also be used by nonathletes who
are recovering from illness, accident, or surgery.

ARTHRITIS WATER THERAPY If the pain of arthritis prevents you from doing most exercise programs, try Arthritis
Water Therapy. The gentle exercises offered here can reduce
the swelling, pain, and inflammation of arthritic joints.

PRENATAL WATERPOWER This program is tailored to meet
your needs during pregnancy. Use the bathtub exercises in
the Prenatal Waterpower chapter as a gentle introduction to

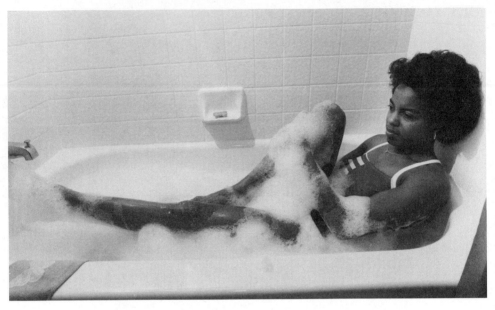

Evelyn Ashford exercising in water during pregnancy.

water exercise. Use the pool exercises for a more vigorous workout that doesn't cause you to bounce or overheat. Remember, always get your doctor's approval before beginning any prenatal exercise routine.

Even if you are not pregnant, there are other uses for Prenatal Waterpower: If you can't leave home, or if you're afraid of water but you've always wanted to have the fun you see others having in water, fill your bathtub and enjoy the pleasurable movements of this program.

THE HOT TUB WORKOUT The hot tub is another soothing place to introduce yourself to water exercise if you are afraid of water. It's also a good way to start if you've been inactive for a long time and want to ease into a program, or if you don't have access to a swimming pool. If you travel, your hotel may have a hot tub where you can work out.

SET YOUR GOALS

Before you start your program, make a copy of the workout chart at the end of that chapter. Seal the chart in see-through plastic to take to the pool when you're ready to go.

Also, consider the progress you hope to make over the coming weeks and months of Waterpower. Your goals should include increasing the number of repetitions. The reps suggested in these programs provide a moderate workout. Start with fewer reps if you feel the need; increase the number of reps as you gain strength and fitness. Always, however, do the exercises in the order presented. The sequence of exercises is as important as the movements.

After your workout, relax and ask yourself these questions:

1. At what point or points did I begin to tire?
2. Which exercises were particularly difficult? What might account for the difficulty?
3. Was there pain with any exercise?
4. Could I have put more effort—speed, power, precision—into the exercises?

The answers to these questions will help you plan your next water workout. Modify difficult exercises and those that cause pain by moving slowly through a narrower range of motion than is seen in the photos or by doing fewer reps. Decide what level of effort you want to commit to the workout. Change your mind only if you encounter pain or unaccountable fatigue.

WATERPOWER PROGRAM GUIDE

Fitness Level	Goals	Waterpower Program
Beginner		
Inactive for many years	Increased strength	Water Stretch
Overweight	Increased balance	The Hot Tub Workout
Afraid of water	Increased flexibility	Prenatal Waterpower

continued on page 10

WATERPOWER PROGRAM GUIDE continued

Fitness Level	Goals	Waterpower Program
Fitness Enthusiast Conditioning program in progress	Improved cardiovascular endurance	Basic Water Workout
	Increased muscular strength	Warm up or warm down with Water Stretch
	Weight control	
Training Athlete All sports	Skill development	Basic Water Workout
	Superior cardiovascular endurance	Water Aerobics
	Superior muscular strength	Sport-Specific Exercises
	Increased flexibility	Warm-down with Water Stretch
Injured Athlete	Retain top level of conditioning	Water Rehabilitation
	Accelerate healing time	Sport-Specific Exercises
	Quickly return to sport with little loss of skill or fitness	Water Stretch
Back Patient Post-Surgical Patient, recovering from accident or illness	Regain strength, balance	Water Stretch
	Increase flexibility	Water Rehabilitation
	Regain coordination, mobility	
Pregnant Woman	Retain muscular strength	Prenatal Waterpower
	Control weight gain	
	Increase abdominal strength	
	Practice deep breathing	
Arthritis Patient		Arthritis Water Therapy

KNOW YOUR BODY

Muscles make up much of the body's weight: approximately 40 percent in men, 30 percent in women. When they contract, they cause movement. Muscles that bend a limb at a joint when they contract are called flexors. Muscles straightening a limb at a joint are called extensors. If the limb is moved away from the midline of the body, an abductor is at work; if the limb is brought toward the midline, adductors are responsible.

All muscles can only pull or relax; they cannot push. Thus back and forth movements of the arms, legs, jaws, or eyes are only possible because muscles work in synchronized pairs—when one contracts, the one opposing it relaxes. The muscles executing the actual movement are known as prime movers or agonists. As the prime movers contract, the opposing muscle group, the antagonists, must relax to allow movement to occur. Then the prime movers must relax as the antagonist contracts in its turn.

These antagonistic muscle pairs maintain a specific ratio of strength and flexibility to each other. If that ratio is thrown out of balance by training or stretching just one of the muscles in a pair, you produce inefficiency and the potential for injury. Therefore it is extremely important to exercise both muscles of each antagonistic pair: quadriceps/hamstrings, thigh adductors/abductors, biceps/triceps, and so forth.

When you exercise on land, you contend with gravity's one-way pull, but when you exercise in water, you must overcome resistance in all directions of movement, allowing you simultaneously to strengthen agonist and antagonist in each muscle pair. For example, when you perform a bicep curl in the weight room, the bicep muscle powerfully contracts to lift up the weight against gravity's force. As you lower the weight, the bicep is again working even as it lengthens to the starting position. To keep the balance in the bicep/tricep muscle pair, you must next perform a separate exercise specifically for the tricep. But in water, you can strengthen both the bicep and

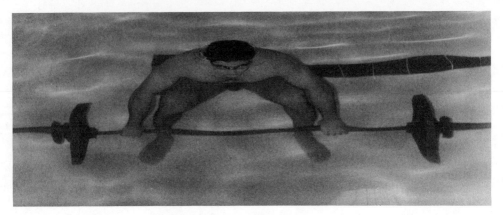

Water supports a lifter as he practices.

the tricep with the same arm curl, for you meet resistance to your movement in both directions of the exercise.

The basic muscle groups are shown in the muscle chart on pages 16–17. If you successfully strengthen these large groups, other minor muscle groups will grow stronger in the process. In each exercise in *The Waterpower Workout*, the prime muscle movers are listed in order of importance, followed by the secondary muscle movers, also in order of importance.

CHOOSING A POOL

Check your potential pool's schedule. Make sure there is an adult swim time, during which you can use the pool without interference from lap-swimmers, children, or divers.

Ideally, the pool you choose for your water training should be no more than 10 to 15 minutes from home or from your work place. The locker room should be inviting, clean, and comfortable. If your "home" pool is easily accessible, and if you look forward to its surroundings, you'll go more often than if it's unattractive or a long drive away.

After you've found your "home" pool, you may be tempted to stop your search for good locations for water training. But that "home" pool may unexpectedly close for cleaning or the schedule may change, interrupting your ideal training time. You should have options, so locate at least two other possible sites for water exercise. The schools near your home may have indoor or outdoor pools that are available to the public for certain hours. If you live near a lake, find a safe point of entry where you can train in chest-deep water. If you live near the ocean, notice which beaches have the calmest surf. You will be able to do most of your exercises there when the waves aren't rough.

When you travel, try to stay at a hotel or motel that has a pool and use it.

SELECTING A SUIT

When you choose your Waterpower suit, think **function not fashion.** Your suit must support you as you jump, sprint, and bounce. Therefore choose a training suit that fits you snugly but stretches comfortably without restricting your movements.

MEN: Select a suit with a drawstring so you can tie it securely around your waist during the jumping portions of your program.

WOMEN: Select a one-piece suit that will adequately support your breasts.

EXTRA EQUIPMENT

If you want to swim laps before or after your water workout, you should use goggles. Goggles not only protect your eyes from the chemicals in the pool water, but also dramatically improve your underwater vision. When you can see clearly, you feel more at ease in what could otherwise seem like an alien environment.

If you want to add workload to your legs during kicking exercises, you can try wearing fins. Kick easily at first or you may strain your hip flexors (groin muscles).

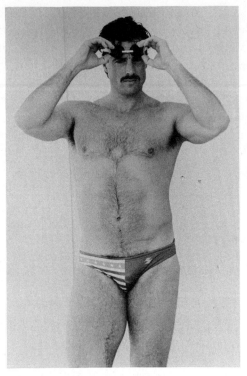

*Goggles help Mac Wilkins see more
clearly if he goes underwater.*

If your program includes sport-specific exercises, take the appropriate equipment to the pool with you: an old baseball bat, tennis racket, football, basketball, or golf club.

If you aren't a strong swimmer, but want to try assisted-swimming devices, begin by using a kickboard to kick around from the shallow end of the pool to the deep end and back.

Back patients can decompress their lower backs while swimming in a controlled posture, using a Perry Flotation Belt coupled with the Perry-Band, a tether that lets you swim in place. Similarly, the Greenberg Float Coat can be used to swim backstroke in place. Explanations of these devices appear later in the book.

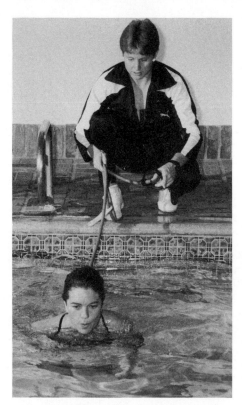

Dr. Vicky Vodon supervises Lynda Huey's water running.

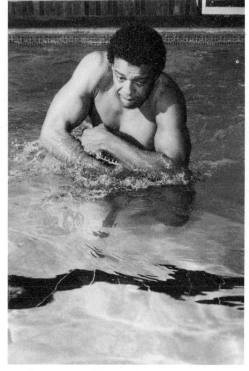

Bernie Casey tightly grips the football and runs hard against water's resistance.

BASIC MUSCLE GROUPS (front)

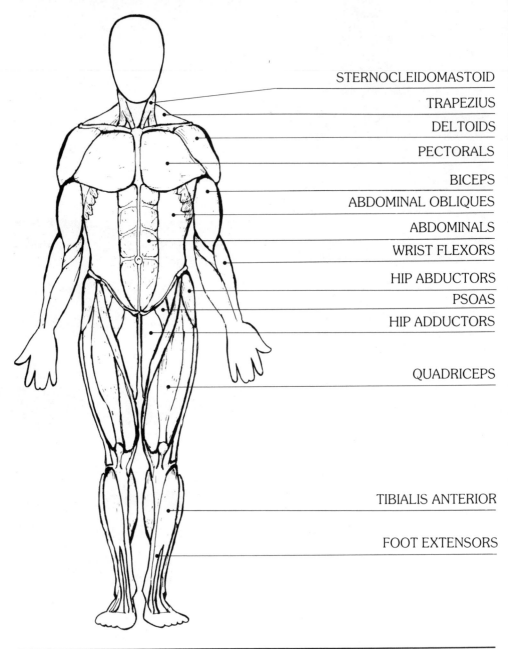

STERNOCLEIDOMASTOID

TRAPEZIUS

DELTOIDS

PECTORALS

BICEPS

ABDOMINAL OBLIQUES

ABDOMINALS

WRIST FLEXORS

HIP ABDUCTORS

PSOAS

HIP ADDUCTORS

QUADRICEPS

TIBIALIS ANTERIOR

FOOT EXTENSORS

BASIC MUSCLE GROUPS (back)

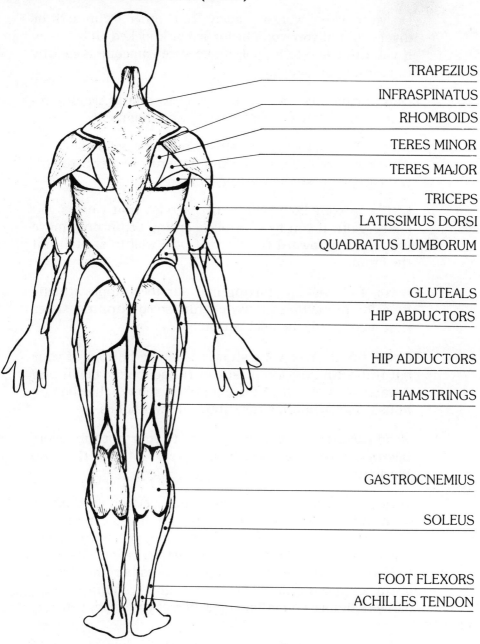

TRAPEZIUS

INFRASPINATUS

RHOMBOIDS

TERES MINOR

TERES MAJOR

TRICEPS

LATISSIMUS DORSI

QUADRATUS LUMBORUM

GLUTEALS

HIP ABDUCTORS

HIP ADDUCTORS

HAMSTRINGS

GASTROCNEMIUS

SOLEUS

FOOT FLEXORS

ACHILLES TENDON

SAFETY TIPS

- Do your water workout away from other swimmers or divers so that you won't be jostled or knocked off balance. If you are alone in a pool, make sure someone is nearby in case of emergency.

- Don't drink alcohol before a water workout. Alcohol impairs your balance, coordination, and judgment.

- Wait at least 2 to 3 hours after a big meal before starting a hard workout. If your workout is gentle (Water Stretch), you can decrease the waiting time to 1 hour.

- Listen to your body. Stop any exercise that causes you sharp pain. If you feel a muscle cramp beginning, move immediately toward the nearest pool wall to stretch out the cramp.

- If you feel blisters starting on your toes, apply athletic tape for protection or wear white-soled running shoes that won't scuff the pool bottom.

- Cover the floor of your shower and the bottom of your bathtub with nonskid plastic or rubber before beginning a water workout. If you use a public shower that has no nonskid protection, wear rubber shower shoes.

- Read the precautions posted next to your hot tub before beginning the exercises in Chapter 11, "The Hot Tub Workout."

- Always use the "buddy system" whenever you exercise in open water—river, bay, ocean, or lake. If you can't find a friend to join you, have someone watch you from shore. If you aren't familiar with the water's currents, the surface and texture of the bottom, or possible underwater obstacles, ask a local resident or lifeguard about possible dangers **before** you enter the water. If you wish, you can modify some of your exercises, working against the current to make them more difficult. In rocky areas, wear an old pair of athletic shoes to protect your feet.

• Do consider joining a class to learn to swim. You will be able to round out your water workouts by doing laps, and you will feel safer each time you enter the water.

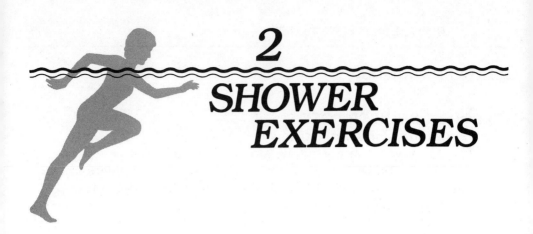

2
SHOWER
EXERCISES

The wonders of water can work for you even when you cannot make it to a swimming pool or spa. You can do these four exercises in your home shower. In the morning these exercises will help you start your day feeling more vital and full of energy. After a tiring day they enable you to relax and release tensions. On a day when you don't have time to do any other form of exercise, these four stretches will help you maintain flexibility and ease the strain of inactivity.

The shower exercises also serve as an excellent warm-up and cool-down for any of the water exercise programs.

SHOWER WARM-UP

Exercise 1 SHOWER POSE
Latissimus dorsi, hamstrings

Place your hands on the side of the shower stall and position your body so that warm spray hits your shoulders and back. Ease your body gently down between the arms, stretching your shoulder joints, as in photo 1. Hold this position while you breathe deeply five times.

Photo 1

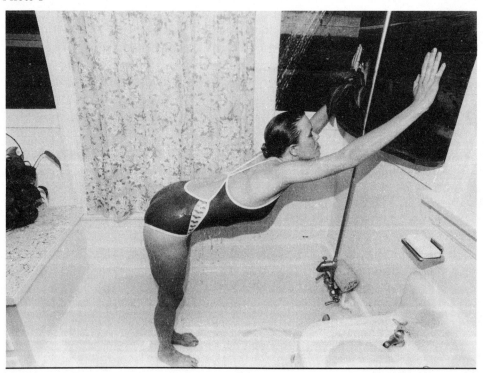

Exercise 2 HAMSTRING STRETCH

Hamstrings, quadratus lumborum

With the shower's water running down your back, place your right foot flat on the wall of the shower stall, as in photo 2. Lean forward from the hips and move your chest slightly toward your right thigh. Place your hands comfortably on your foot, ankle, or shin. Relax your neck by letting your head fall forward. Breathe deeply and hold the position five breaths. Repeat with the left leg. As you learn to enjoy this stretch, you may want to hold the position longer.

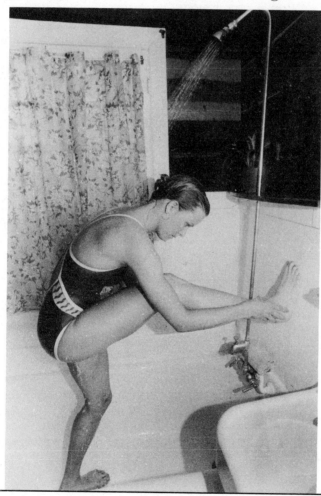

Photo 2

SHOWER COOL-DOWN

Exercise 3 CLASP-HANDS-BEHIND-BACK STRETCH
Rhomboids, delts, pecs

Stand with your back to the spray. Interlace your fingers behind your back so that water strikes you between your shoulder blades (photo 3). Pull your shoulders back, squeezing your shoulder blades together. Breathe deeply five times as you hold the position. Relax and repeat.

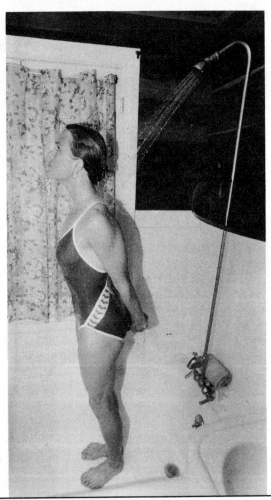

Photo 3

Exercise 4 RAG DOLL

Trapezius, hamstrings, gastrocs, quadratus lumborum

Facing away from the shower, relax your neck and bring your chin to your chest, stretching the muscles of your neck and upper back (photo 4A). Let the warm water pound against your upper body as you breathe deeply five times.

Now bend your knees, bend forward at the hips, and let your body hang as in photo 4B. Position yourself so that the water sprays your lower back. Be sure your eyes look straight down at the floor, not behind you. Otherwise water runs into your nose.

Before leaving the shower, lower the water temperature to complete your cool-down.

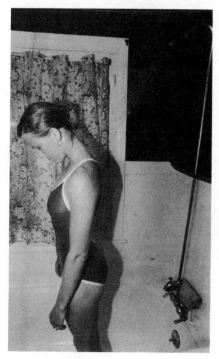

Photo 4A

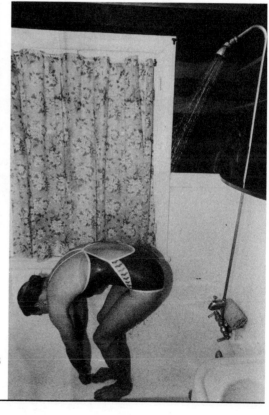

Photo 4B

SHOWER WORKOUT

SHOWER WARM-UP

Exercise 1 SHOWER POSE
5 breaths

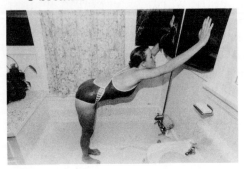

Exercise 2 HAMSTRING STRETCH

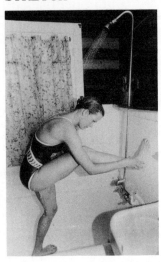

SHOWER COOL-DOWN

Exercise 3 CLASP-HANDS-BEHIND-BACK STRETCH
5 breaths

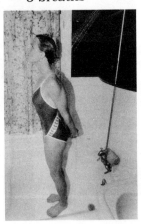

Exercise 4 RAG DOLL
5 breaths
Bend knees, bend forward—5 breaths

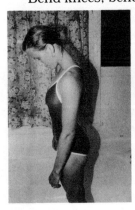
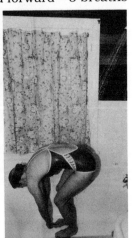

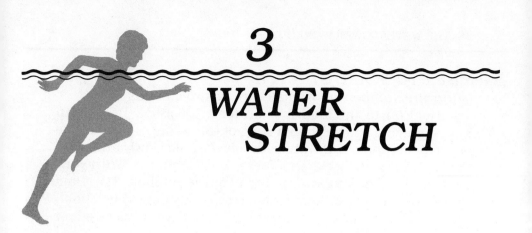

3
WATER
STRETCH

You can move through this beginning program in approximately 10 minutes, or you can take your own sweet time. You can stretch every day or only twice a week. You can stretch with a partner or you can stretch alone. Just remember that if Water Stretch is your first step in becoming fit, you should continue this gentle regimen for at least two weeks before attempting a more strenuous water workout.

These exercises should be done in sequence 1 through 8. Don't avoid any movement that might seem too difficult at first. Do each stretch as best you can. If you experience difficulty, concentrate on breathing slowly and deeply. Ease away from the stretch on an inhale; stretch further on the exhale.

As soon as you enter the pool, the magic of water begins to work for you. Water's buoyancy counteracts much of gravity's force, increasing joint space in the ankles, knees, hips, and between the vertebrae of the spine. Stretching the joints and the surrounding muscles to the maximum is thus easier in water than on land. Water's buoyancy also reduces the stiffness and muscle discomfort you might feel during a stretch on land. Further, water's soothing quality relaxes you, easing away both physical and mental tension.

If you're feeling stiff before Water Stretch, begin with the added help of hot water and Shower Warm-ups (see pages 22–23). End with Shower Cool-downs (see pages 24–25).

Exercise 1 TUCK AND STRETCH
Quatratus lumborum, hamstrings, gastrocnemius

Hold on to the ladder or gutter at poolside. Bend both knees, placing your feet on a rung of the ladder or on the side of the pool (photo 1A). Inhale deeply. Exhale slowly and completely relax your neck, shoulders, back, and legs. With your next exhalation, slowly straighten your legs (photo 1B). Hold this position for five long slow breaths, keeping your shoulders and arms as relaxed as possible. Bend your knees on an inhale, returning to the starting position. Repeat.

Photo 1a

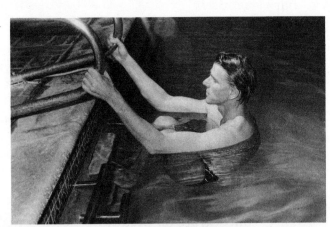

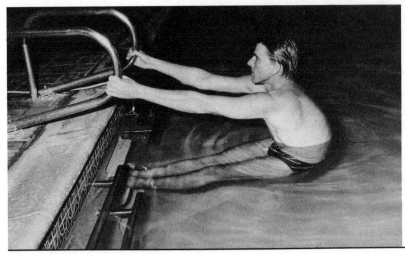

Photo 1b

Exercise 2 SHOULDER STRETCH

Latissimus dorsi, infraspinatus, teres major and minor

Bend and raise your right elbow. Place your right hand flat on your back between your shoulder blades. Grasp your right elbow with your left hand and gently pull the elbow to the left, stretching the muscles of the right shoulder as in photo 2. (This photo and others to come was shot on land so you can see more clearly what would be the body's position underwater.) By slightly bending your knees, you can avoid the tendency to arch your back, which compresses your lumbar vertebrae. Bend your knees further until your chin is just above the water level and your shoulders are submerged. Breathe deeply five times as you relax and allow the muscles to stretch. Repeat with the left arm.

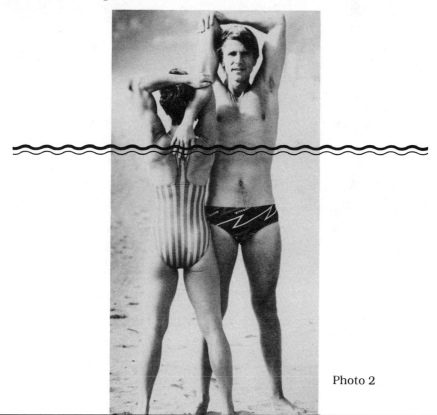

Photo 2

Exercise 3 TRIANGLE
Lats, gluteus medius, abdominal obliques

Stand in chest-deep water with feet shoulder-width apart. Lift your left arm straight up and over your head, letting your right hand slide down your right leg under the water (photo 3). The hips face forward throughout this stretch. Do not twist to the side. Breathe deeply as you feel this stretch relax the muscles from the area of the hip up through the arm and shoulder. Repeat with the right arm. A partner can help you maintain your position, preventing twisting in the Triangle.

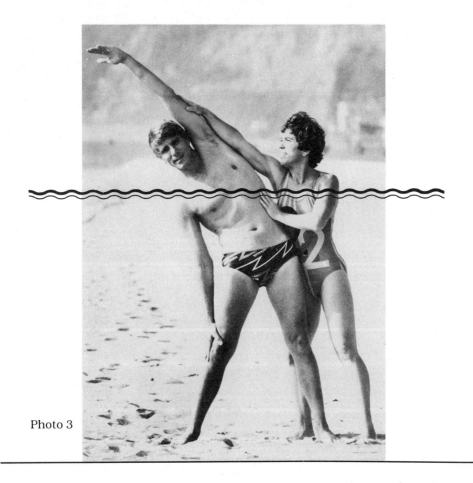

Photo 3

Exercise 4 KNEE PULL STRETCH

Quadratus lumborum, hamstrings, gluts

Stand on your right foot in chest-deep water. Clasp both hands around your left knee and pull toward your chest (photo 4). Hold this position as you squeeze your knee next to the body. Breathe deeply. The water will support you throughout this balancing stretch.

Repeat with the right knee.

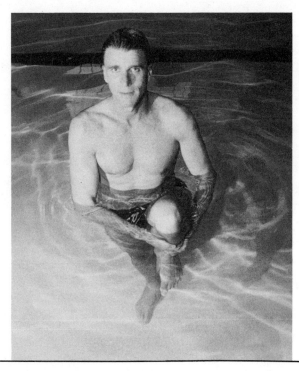

Photo 4

Exercise 5 CRESCENT MOON

Lats, upper quadriceps, gastrocnemius, abdominals

Move into waist-deep water. Lift both arms straight over-head as you lunge forward into the position in photo 5. Your right knee will be directly over the right foot. Both feet point straight ahead. Tuck your tailbone down. Now look up at your hands. Although this position would be quite difficult to maintain on land, the water assists and supports you, making Crescent Moon easy. Breathe deeply as you hold the position. Slowly lower yourself deeper into the water, increasing the stretch in the right upper quads and lower abdominals. This stretch protects against groin injuries.

Repeat with the left leg.

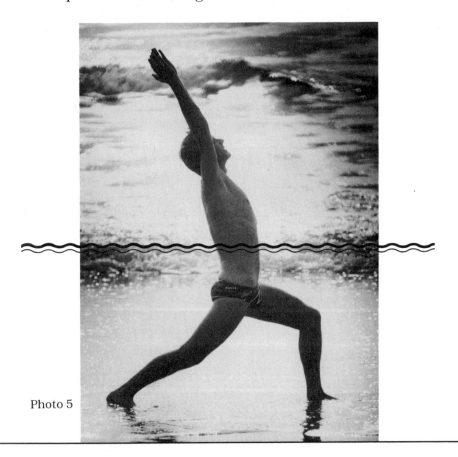

Photo 5

Exercise 6 QUAD STRETCH
Quads, lower abdominals

Stand on your left foot. Bend your right knee and hold your right foot behind you with your right hand. Slowly pull the right heel toward the buttocks, as in photo 6. Never force a stretch if there is pain. Stretch only to the point of discomfort, ease back a bit, and hold the position until the muscles have relaxed and lengthened. Deep breathing facilitates the stretching and balancing processes.

Repeat with the left leg.

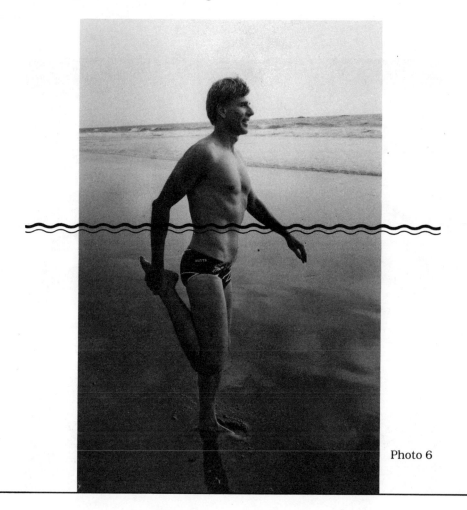

Photo 6

Exercise 7 GROIN STRETCH

Upper quads, lower abdominals, pectorals

From the Quad Stretch position (Exercise 6), move directly into the Groin Stretch by maintaining the hold on your ankle and letting your leg swing back as you lift your foot (photo 7). The hips face forward throughout this stretch. Hold your free arm up in front of you for balance. If this balance is difficult for you, start with your free hand touching the side of the pool.

Repeat for other leg.

Photo 7

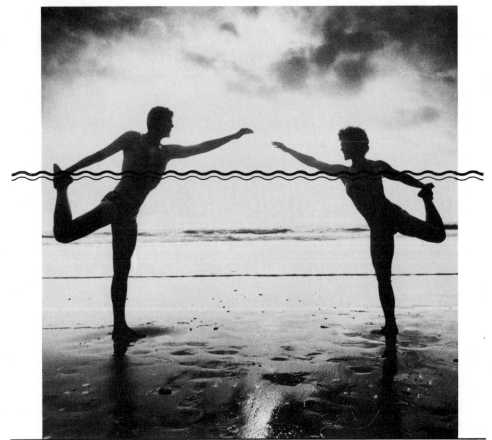

Exercise 8 HAMSTRING STRETCH

Hamstrings, quadratus lumborum

Face the side of the pool. Lift your right leg onto the railing, gutter, or side of the pool. If this is too difficult, start with the knee slightly bent. With an inhalation, lift your chest; with an exhalation, lower your head and chest down toward your leg (photo 8A). Breathe deeply five times as you allow the hamstring and lower back muscles to relax. Repeat with the left leg.

Photo 8A

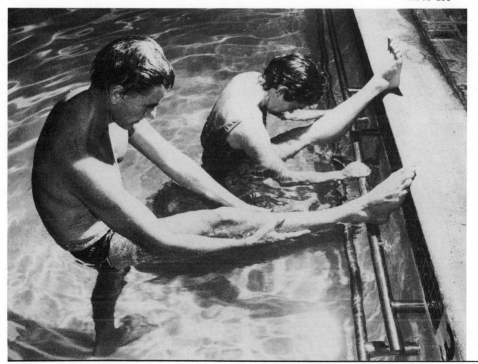

continued on page 36

Exercise 8 HAMSTRING STRETCH continued

If you are in water that has no supporting structure nearby, you can stretch your hamstrings as in photo 8B. Step forward with your left foot, keeping both knees straight. Both feet point straight ahead. Place your hands on your left knee for support, then lean forward, stretching the left hamstring.

Repeat with the right leg.

Photo 8B

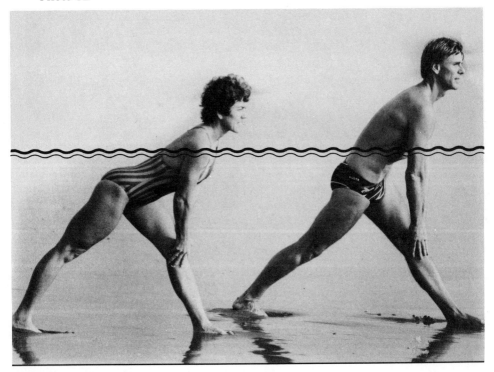

IMPROVING YOUR WATER STRETCH

After you have finished these exercises for the first time, look again at the photo illustrations in this chapter. You may not have achieved the maximum stretch in these positions. In trying to do so during your next workout, don't force your stretch. If you feel pain, you have stretched too far. Pull back slightly and hold the stretch where you feel comfortable and can breathe easily. **Don't bounce.** Holding a steady stretch is more effective. Breathe deeply and slowly. As you breathe and hold the position you will notice that your body tends to relax as you exhale, allowing you to ease more deeply into your stretch.

You will find that Water Stretch quickly becomes a pleasant habit. You can stretch when you're energetic—and stay energetic. You can stretch when you're tired—and grow no more tired. Water stretching can be your total fitness program or your warm-up or warm-down for more vigorous programs, such as the Basic Waterpower Workout in the next chapter.

WATER STRETCH WORKOUT

SHOWER WARM-UP (Optional)

SHOWER POSE
5 breaths

HAMSTRING STRETCH
5 breaths

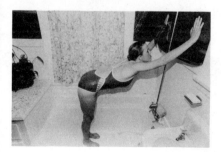
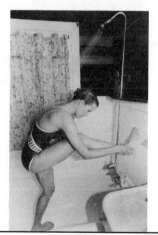

continued on page 38

WATER STRETCH WORKOUT continued

1. TUCK AND STRETCH 2 reps of 5 breaths

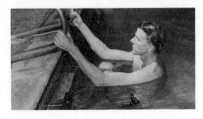 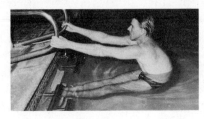

2. SHOULDER STRETCH
5 breaths each side

3. TRIANGLE
5 breaths each side

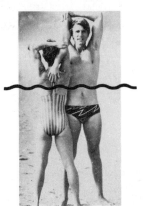 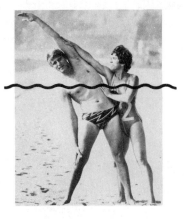

4. KNEE-PULL STRETCH 5 breaths each side

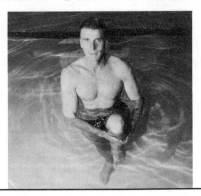

5. *CRESCENT MOON*
5 breaths each side

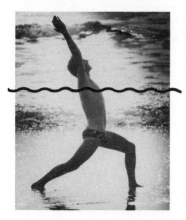

6. *QUAD STRETCH*
5 breaths each side

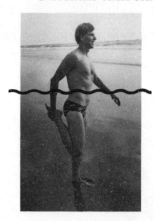

7. *GROIN STRETCH* 5 breaths each side

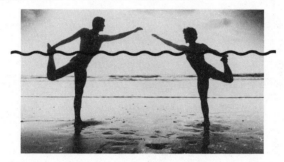

8. *HAMSTRING STRETCH* 5 breaths each side

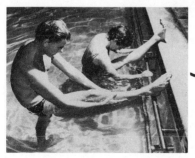
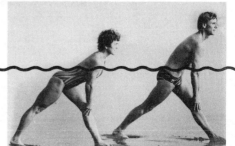

continued on page 40

WATER STRETCH WORKOUT continued

SHOWER COOL-DOWN (Optional)

CLASP-HANDS-BEHIND-BACK STRETCH
 5 breaths

RAG DOLL
 5 breaths
 Bend knees, Bend forward—5 breaths

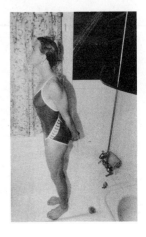

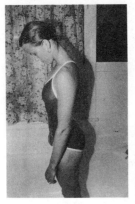

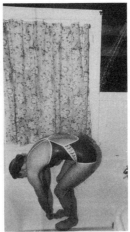

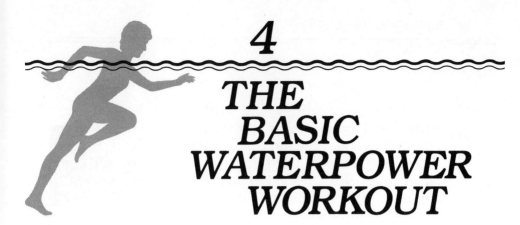

4

THE BASIC WATERPOWER WORKOUT

On land you would need a lengthy warm-up stretch before attempting the jumps and sprints to follow. But, because the water's resistance doesn't allow the body to work as fast as on land, and because the water provides a cushion for the explosive moves to come, there's much less risk of injury and thus less need for stretching before beginning the Basic Waterpower Workout. Still, if you feel more comfortable with a warm-up stretch, do shower warm-ups or Water Stretch before you begin.

The 20 exercises take about 45 minutes to complete. This program provides you with a solid aerobic workout rounded out with exercises specifically for your abdominals, arms, and legs. End with a pleasant shower cool-down.

For maximum benefit, keep the following tips in mind:

- When you're ready to enter the pool, move away from the wall to chest-deep water.

- In-between exercises 1 through 11, keep moving by bouncing or running in place to keep your heart rate up. Bouncing is a rhythmic up and down movement that is even easier to do in water than on land. When you bounce or jump, inhale at the height of the jump and exhale at the point nearest the water. This prevents you from accidentally swallowing water.

- If you've been conditioning with Water Stretch for a while, and are moving on for the greater challenge of the Basic Waterpower Workout, ease yourself into it by doing half of the recommended repetitions. Warm up and down with Water Stretch. Allow your body at least one month to adapt to this new workload before gradually increasing your reps until you reach the number of reps suggested on The Basic Waterpower Workout chart.

- Use the Basic Waterpower Workout to maintain and increase strength for your sport. If you can't or don't feel like making your regular basketball game or track workout, stay in competitive shape by doing this overall workout along with Sport-Specific Water Training drills. In this way you will do a solid cardiovascular workout while the sport-specific exercises will help you maintain your sport skills.

- For an even more rigorous training program, use the Basic Water Workout along with Water Aerobics and Sport-Specific exercises. This combination supplies enough cardiovascular and muscular workload for even the most serious of athletes.

Exercise 1 BOUNCING
Quadriceps, hamstrings, gastrocnemius, feet extensors

Begin bouncing with your feet comfortably apart, toes pointed straight ahead. Bend your knees as you come down and straighten them as you rise, 25 times.

First Variation
Deltoids, quads, gluteals, gastrocs, feet extensors

Raise both arms straight over your head as you bounce

as high as you can (photo 1). Reach forcefully toward the ceiling on each bounce. Each time you land, let your hands drop to your ears. Repeat 10 times.

Second Variation
Gastrocs, feet flexors and extensors
    Now straighten your knees and drop your arms comfortably to your sides. Continue the bouncing movements using only the feet and calf muscles for upward thrust, 25 times.

Total—60

Keep bouncing or running in place. Time—1:00

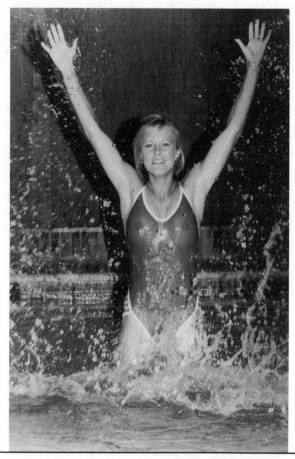

Photo 1

Exercise 2 JUMPING, NO ARMS

Abdominals, abdominal obliques, quads, gluts, hamstrings, gastrocs, feet

In this exercise, your stomach and leg muscles rather than your arms will direct the movement of the body. With your ankles together, hold your arms tightly against your sides and begin jumping forward and backward, 15 times. More coordination is required when you try this same exercise jumping side-to-side, 15 times. Count 1 each time you complete a front-back cycle. Count 1 for each side-to-side cycle.

Total—30

Time—1:00

From here through Exercise 10, only primary muscle movers are listed. Gastrocs and feet muscles are secondary movers in all exercises where the feet touch the bottom of the pool. Abdominal muscles act as secondary movers in stabilizing the body in nearly all exercises.

Exercise 3 LUNGES

Quads, hamstrings, abdominals, deltoids, gluts

Bend your right knee and place your right foot a full stride in front of your left foot. Your left arm should be forward for counterbalance (photo 3). Jump up and switch arm and leg positions so that the left leg is now forward and the right arm is forward. Repeat 25 times. Again, this exercise has two parts, so each right-left cycle should be counted as only 1 repetition.   Total—25

Time—1:00

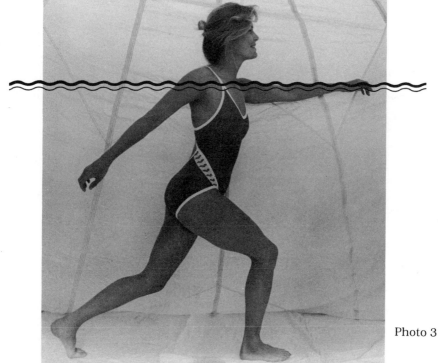

Photo 3

Exercise 4 HITCH KICKS

Quads, psoas, abdominals, delts

Lift your right leg straight out in front of you while you continue bouncing on your left foot. Reach forward with your left arm for counterbalance (photo 4). Jump up and switch arm and leg positions so that the left leg is now held straight in front of you and the right arm is forward. Repeat 15 cycles.   Total—15

Keep bouncing or running in place.   Time—:30

Exercise 5 ROCKING HORSE

Pectoralis, lats, quads, hamstrings, abdominals

Continue working in the middle of the pool, in chest-deep water. Bounce on your right foot and hold your left leg straight in front of you. Extend your arms straight out to your

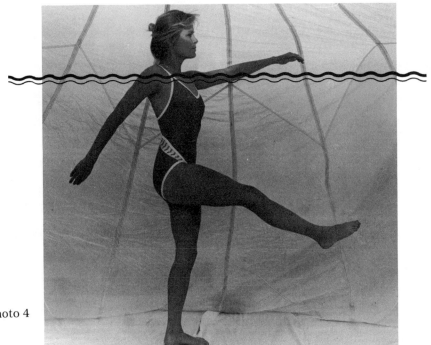

Photo 4

sides (photo 5A). Rock forward onto your left foot and swing your right leg straight behind you. At the same time, sweep both arms through the water to position 5B. Continue rocking forward onto the left foot and backward onto the right foot, pulling your arms forward and backward on each rock. Repeat 15 cycles. Reverse foot positions (right foot forward and left foot back) 15 more cycles.   Total—30
Time—1:15

Photo 5A

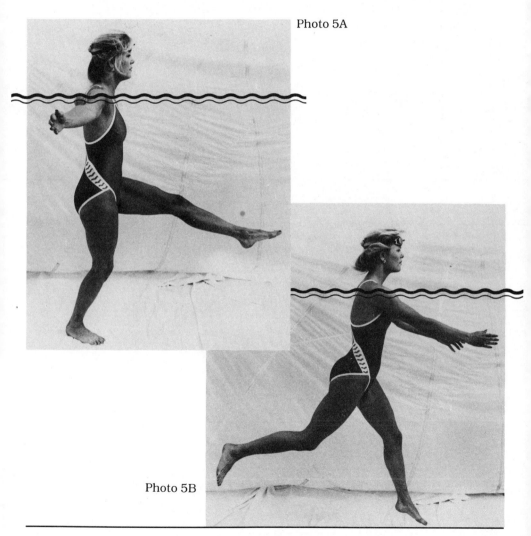

Photo 5B

Exercise 6 STRADDLE JUMPS
Adductors, abductors, quads

Begin jumping with your feet together and your hands on your hips. Jump up, open your legs sideways, and bring them back together before you land, 15 times (photo 6).

The variation that follows is easier to do. Continue jumping but this time with your feet shoulder-width apart. Jump up, bringing your feet together at the top of your jump. Land with your feet back in their open position, 15 reps.

Continue bouncing.

Total—30

Time—1:00

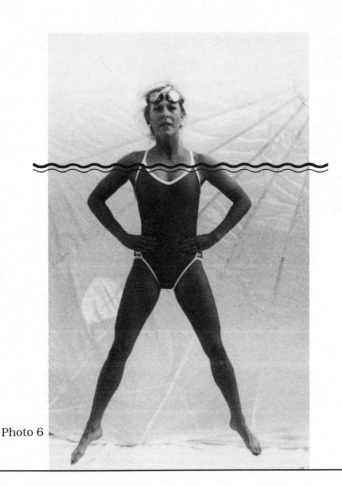

Photo 6

Exercise 7 FROG JUMPS

Abdominals, quads, psoas

Bouncing in place on both feet, jump high and pull both knees toward your chest. Your arms can remain loosely at your sides, helping to initiate each jump. Keep on with this for 25 straight jumps. If you wish to increase the difficulty of this exercise, hold your arms overhead as in photo 7. Notice the water turbulence created as Marlene lifts her knees.

Total—25
Time—:45

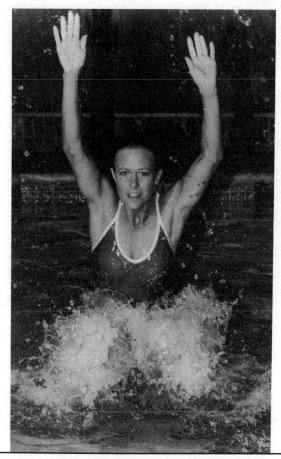

Photo 7

Exercise 8 JUMP AND SPRINT

Quads, hamstrings, delts, biceps, gluts

Begin by reaching with straight arms toward the ceiling as you jump in place five times (photo 8A). Directly off the fifth jump, begin sprinting in place (photo 8B). Sprint for about 10 seconds. Alternate jumping and sprinting in this manner for 1 to 2 minutes.

Continue bouncing.   Time—1–2 mins.

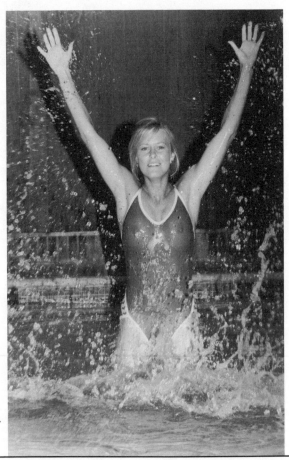

Photo 8A

Exercise 9 INTERVALS

Biceps, quads, hamstrings, gluts

With your arms comfortably at your sides, bounce slowly in place. Then, off the bounce, sprint in place for 30 seconds. During sprinting you will use your arms to power your legs, as in photo 8B. Now bounce gently for a 30-second recovery, then sprint again. Alternate these work bouts and recovery periods.

Vary the length of your sprint intervals each day to keep this exercise fresh. For example, you may wish to run "step-ups" (15 secs., 30 secs., 45 secs., 60 secs.) or "break-downs" (60 secs., 45 secs., 30 secs., 15 secs.) Or you may wish to run three to five intervals of the same length of time. Just be sure you make your recovery period equal to the length of time of your workout. If there's no clock at your pool, count the seconds yourself.   Time—5–8 mins.

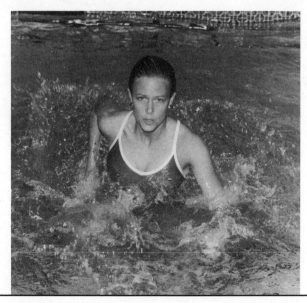

Photo 8B

Exercise 10 WATER TRIPPING

Quads, hamstrings, abdominals

Run from one side of the pool to the other and back in chest-deep water. Drive your arms powerfully forward and backward under the water to aid the movement. Feet should point straight ahead while running.

After two laps, gradually slow down and change from a run to a two-footed jump. Continue crossing the pool with:

- 2-footed jumps forward (photo 10)
- 2-footed jumps backward
- Right foot jumps forward
- Left foot jumps forward
- Right foot jumps backward
- Left foot jumps backward
- Backward running, pulling elbows backward through the water on each stride

Time—3:00

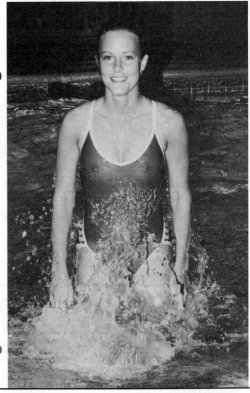

Photo 10

Exercise 11 POOLSIDE FLUTTER KICK
Quads, hamstrings, abdominals, gluts

Turn your back to the wall of the pool and brace yourself with your arms on the edge of the pool. Lift both legs in front of you, bend your knees, and kick in a bicycling movement 25 cycles, counting each time your right knee breaks the surface of the water (photo 11). Next, kick with straight legs for 25 cycles.

Turn over and face the pool's wall. Hold on to the ladder, ledge, or side of the pool, and extend your legs behind you. Your face is out of the water. Bend your knees and kick 25 cycles, letting your feet come out of the water behind you. Then kick with straight legs for 25 cycles.　　　　Total—100

Time—2:00

Photo 11

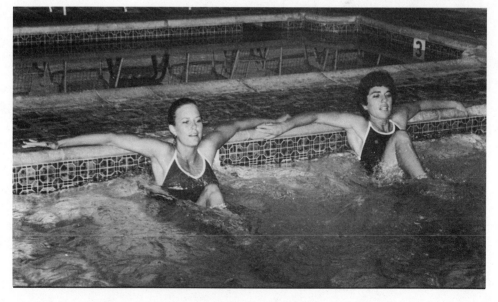

Exercise 12 SCISSORS

Abductors, adductors, abdominals, quads, psoas

Take the position in photo 12 letting your lower back rest against the pool's wall. Extend both your legs straight out in front of you and open them sideways. With a scissors motion, cross and recross them, alternating top leg. Use as much force in closing the legs as you use in opening them. Repeat 15 times.

Total—15

Time—:45

Exercise 13 KNEES TO CHEST TWIST

Abdominal obliques, quads, psoas, adductors

Stay braced at the wall (as above), and squeeze your knees to your chest as tightly as you can. Twist to the right, then to the left (photo 13), 15 times in each direction.

Total—15

Time—:20

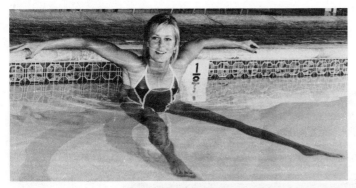

Photo 12

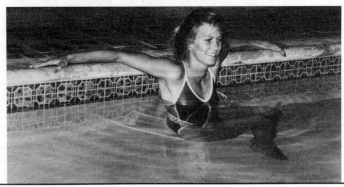

Photo 13

Exercise 14 DIPS

Triceps, forearm flexors and extensors, lats

Stand in chest-deep water facing the side of the pool. Place your hands palms down on the deck. Now jump up and straighten your elbows, supporting yourself as in photo 14A. From this position, bend your knees (so your feet will not touch the pool's bottom) and lower yourself as far as you can without losing control (photo 14B).

If this exercise is too difficult for you, be content for several weeks with merely holding yourself steadily in the starting position. Over the passing weeks of Waterpower, you will be able to dip yourself to the lowest position. Begin with 5 reps, gradually working up to 15.　　　　　Total—15

Time—:40

Photo 14A

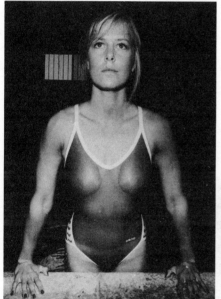

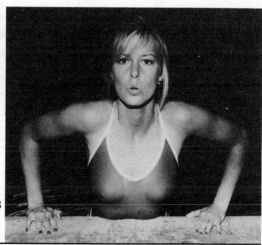

Photo 14B

Exercise 15 PADDLING

Pecs, lats, rhomboids

Now move closer to the middle of the pool. Bend your knees until water covers your shoulders. Cup your hands and extend both arms straight out in front of you with the back of your hands touching each other (photo 15A). Pull your arms through the water until they are straight out from your sides. Now flip your palms to face forward (photo 15B) and sweep your hands to a clap in front of your body. Repeat 15 times.

Photo 15A

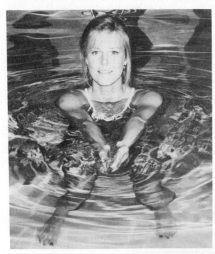

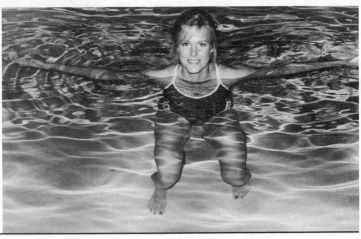

Photo 15B

First Variation
Lats, delts, pecs

Reach your arms straight out in front of your body, hands cupped and facing down (photo 15C). Now pull your arms down past your hips until your hands break the surface of the water behind you (photo 15D). Flip your palms over and pull the arms forward until your cupped hands break the surface of the water in front of you. Repeat 15 times.

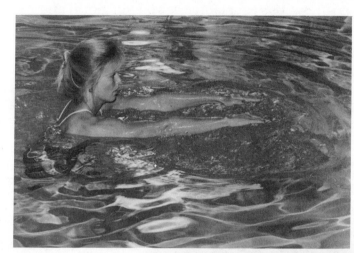

Photo 15C

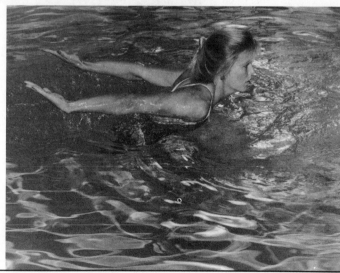

Photo 15D

continued on page 58

Exercise 15 PADDLING continued

Second Variation
Lats, delts

Hold both arms straight out to your sides at shoulder level, palms down (photo 15E). Hands are flat with the fingers held tightly together. Pull the arms down until your hands approach each other behind the buttocks (photo 15F). Without changing your hand position, lift the arms straight back to the starting position. Use equal force as you pull down and lift up. Repeat 15 times.

Third Variation
Lats, delts, pecs

Continue the same up-and-down motion with the arms as in the second variation, but now clap the hands in front of the pubic bone. Repeat 15 times. Total—60
Time—2:30

Photo 15E   Photo 15F

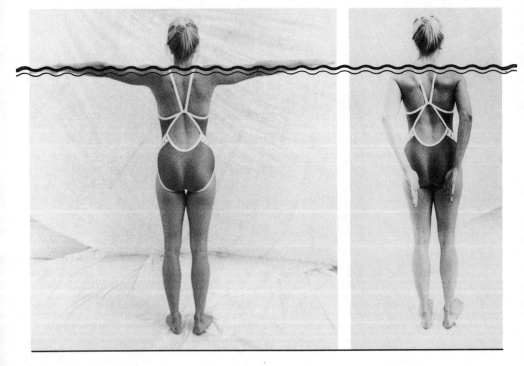

Exercise 16 TWISTER

Lats, abdominal obliques, pecs, quadratus lumborum

Again, bend your knees until water covers your shoulders. Extend your arms at shoulder height directly out from your sides. Palms face forward and fingers are held tightly together. Pivot your feet on the bottom of the pool as you twist your upper body first to the right, then back to the left. Continue twisting, making sure your arms stay at the surface of the water in a straight line (photo 16). Repeat 10 times.

Some who practice Waterpower happily report this exercise causes vertebral self-adjustments; others experience a pleasing massage of the colon.   Total—10

Time—1:00

Photo 16

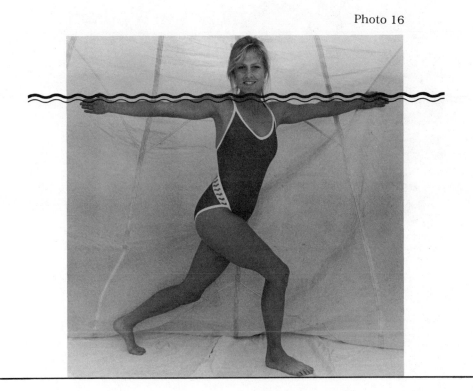

Exercise 17 LATERAL LEG RAISES

Abductors, adductors, gastrocs, abdominals

Look at photo 17A. Take that position at the side of the pool. You will be standing on your toes. Lift your left leg directly to the side (photo 17B), then pull your left leg back to the starting position.

Apply equal force as you lift the leg up and pull it down. Face the opposite direction and repeat on the other leg for 15 reps. Your calves may tire before you complete 15 reps. In that event, come to a flat-footed stance and continue.   Total—30
Time—:45

Photo 17A   Photo 17B

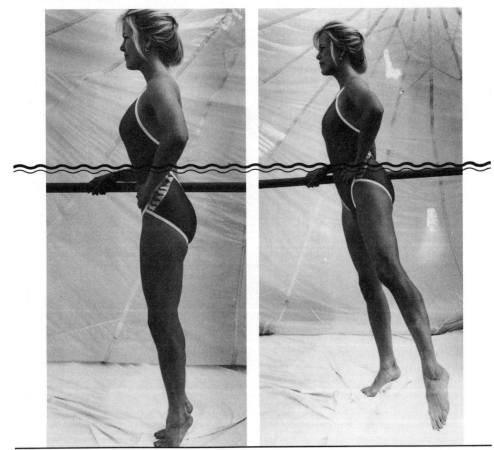

Exercise 18 HAMSTRING CURLS

Hamstrings, quads, gastrocs

Starting at the same position shown in 17A, bring your left heel up toward the left buttock (photo 18), then kick your toes down toward the bottom of the pool. Kick up and down with equal force 15 times. Repeat with the right leg.

Total—30
Time—1:00

Photo 18

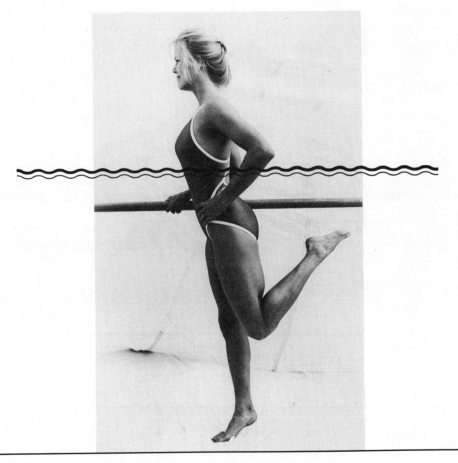

Exercise 19 QUAD EXTENSIONS

Quads, hamstrings, psoas, gastrocs

Maintain the same body position as in Exercise 18, but lift your right knee in front of your body as seen in photo 19A. Kick the lower leg away (photo 19B), then pull it back to the starting position, 15 times. If this position is too difficult for you, lower the right knee partway and kick from that position. Repeat with the left leg 15 times.   Total—30

Time—1:15

Photo 19A   Photo 19B

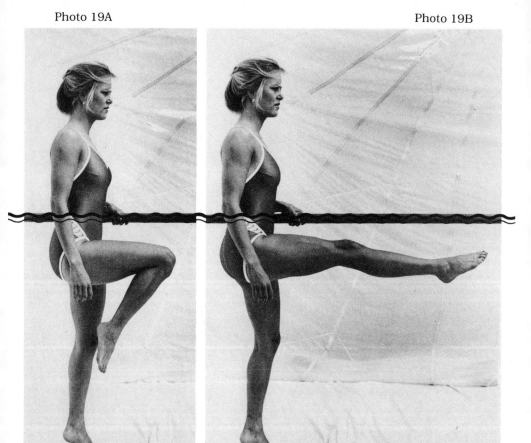

Exercise 20 LEG SWINGS
Abdominals, psoas, quads, hamstrings, gluts, gastrocs

Continue standing tall on your toes. Swing your right leg straight in front of you (photo 20A), then swing it down and to the rear (photo 20B). Swing your leg forward and backward 10 times. Repeat with the left leg.   Total—20

Time—1:20

Now have your cool-down shower.

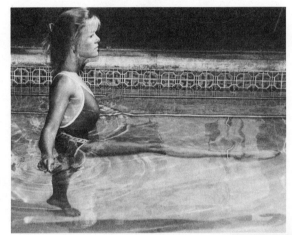

Photo 20A

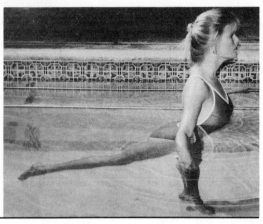

Photo 20B

THE BASIC WATERPOWER WORKOUT

SHOWER WARM-UP (Optional)

SHOWER POSE 5 breaths   *HAMSTRING STRETCH* 5 breaths

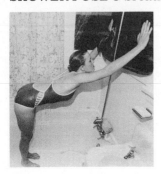   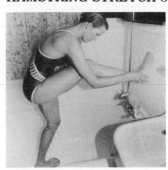

1. *BOUNCING* 25 reps, Hands over head—10 reps
   Straight legs—25 reps

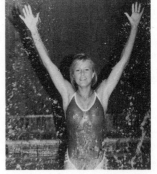

2. *JUMPING, NO ARMS*
   Forward/backward—15 reps
   Side-to-side—15 reps

3. *LUNGES* 25 reps   4. *HITCH KICKS* 15 reps

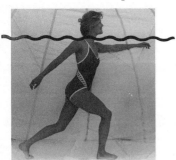   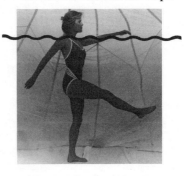

5. *ROCKING HORSE* 15 reps each side

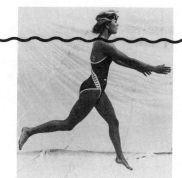

6. *STRADDLE JUMPS*
Feet together—15 reps
Feet apart—15 reps

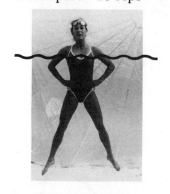

7. *FROG JUMPS*
25 reps

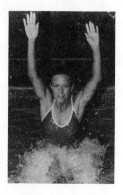

8. *JUMP AND SPRINT*
5 reps

9. *INTERVALS*
30 sec. on/30 sec. off

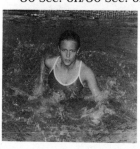

10. *WATER TRIPPING* 3 minutes
2-footed jumps forward
2-footed jumps backward
Right foot jumps forward
Left foot jumps forward
Right foot jumps backward
Left foot jumps backward
Backward running, pulling
   elbows backward

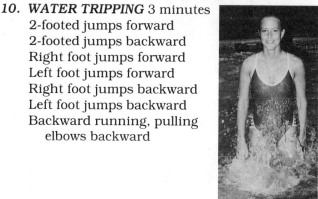

continued on page 66

THE BASIC WATERPOWER WORKOUT continued

11. *POOLSIDE FLUTTER KICK*
Back with bicycle, then straight legs—25 reps each
Front with bent, then straight legs—25 reps each

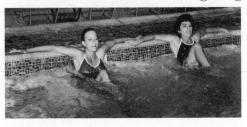

12. *SCISSORS* 15 reps

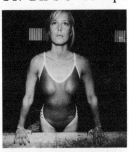

13. *KNEES TO CHEST TWIST*
15 reps each direction

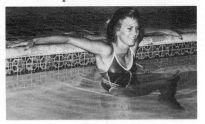

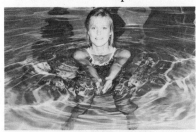

14. *DIPS* 5–15 reps

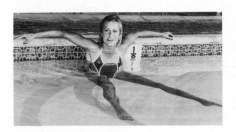

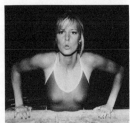

15. *PADDLING*
Lateral—15 reps

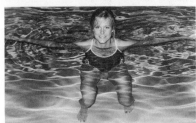

15. *PADDLING continued*

Pull down, lift behind—15 reps   Downward, upward—15 reps

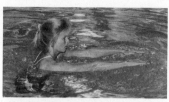

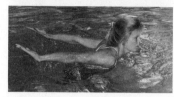

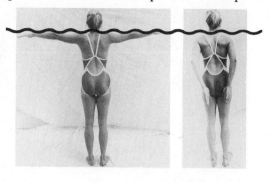

17. *LATERAL LEG RAISES* 15 reps

16. *TWISTER* 10 reps

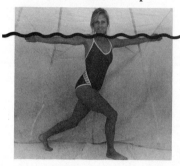

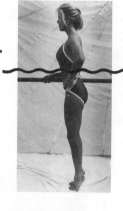

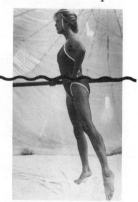

18. *HAMSTRING CURLS*
15 reps each side

19. *QUAD EXTENSIONS* 15 reps each side

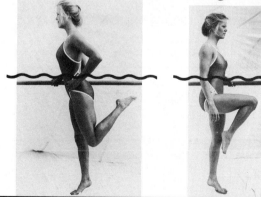

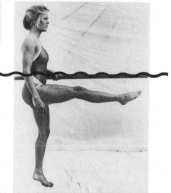

continued on page 68

THE BASIC WATERPOWER WORKOUT continued

20. *LEG SWINGS* 10 reps each side
Bend knees, bend forward—5 breaths

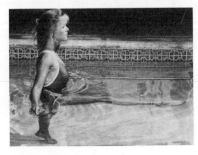 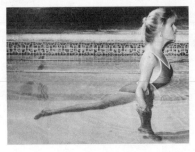

SHOWER COOL-DOWN

CLASP-HANDS-BEHIND-BACK STRETCH
5 breaths

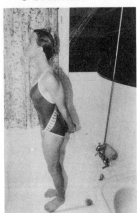

RAG DOLL 5 breaths
Bend Knees, Bend Forward—5 breaths

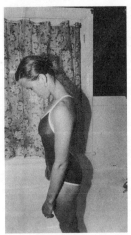 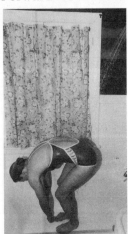

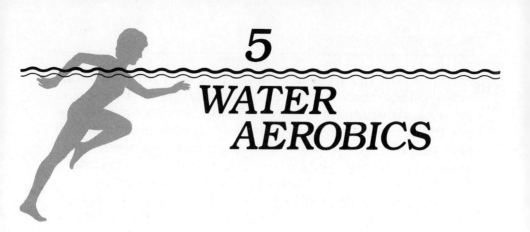

5
WATER AEROBICS

When you're ready to try Water Aerobics for the first time, sit quietly for 10 minutes, then take your pulse this way: Place two fingers over your carotid artery (as seen in photo on page 71) and count the beats you feel there for 30 seconds on your stopwatch. Multiply the number of beats you count by 2 and you have your resting heart rate.

Your **resting heart rate** is an indicator of your fitness level. If you are a well-conditioned athlete, your resting heart rate may be as **low** as 40 or 50 beats per minute. Your heart, like the other muscles of your body, has become more efficient with exercise. A more efficient heart can contract more forcefully each beat, pumping a larger volume of blood each beat. If you are out of condition, your resting heart rate will probably be **higher** than the average resting heart rate, which is 70 beats per minute for men and 80 beats per minute for women. Those of you who have been sedentary for years are probably badly out of condition.

Your **resting heart rate** will increase, becoming your **working heart rate** as you enter the pool and begin Water

Aerobics. The harder you work in the water, the faster your heart will beat, carrying more and more oxygen to the working muscles. (Your ability to transport oxygen is your aerobic capacity.) If you slow down your workout, your heart will also slow its beating. Because of this relationship between workload and heart rate, you can use your **working heart rate** as a precise indicator of the intensity of any exercise session.

To improve the efficiency of your heart—thereby improving your overall fitness level—you must train your heart like any other muscle. You must exercise it. As your heart is exercised it adapts, becoming stronger because of the added work.

How hard must you work your heart? How often? And for how long a time period in order to progress toward this cardiovascular fitness?

Fitness researchers have given us precise guidelines to answer these questions: **Cardiovascular fitness can be improved (the "training effect") by training at least 3 times a week with a working heart rate elevated to 70 to 85 percent of maximum heart rate and kept there, by continuous workload, for at least 20 minutes each training session.**

Your **maximum heart rate** can be determined from a standard formula: 220 minus your age. For example, if you are 30 years old, your predicted maximum heart rate is 220 minus 30, or 190 beats per minute. Once you know your maximum heart rate, compute 70 percent and 85 percent of that number to figure the lower and upper boundaries of your **target heart rate** zone. (See chart on page 72.) It is within that target zone that you must keep your working heart rate for at least 20 minutes each time you do the Water Aerobics program in this chapter.

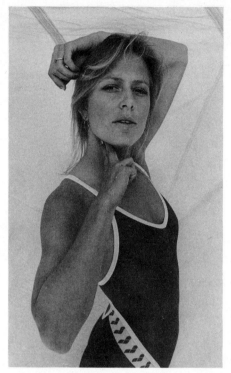

Marlene Harmon takes her pulse.

Remember these essential guidelines when doing Water Aerobics:

- **Frequency**—you must do Water Aerobics at least 3 times a week.

- **Intensity**—you must work hard enough to raise your working heart rate to your target zone (70 to 85 percent of your maximum heart rate).

- **Duration**—you must work within your target zone for at least 20 minutes during each exercise session.

WORKING HEART RATE TARGET ZONES

Women	Age	Minimum	Optimum	Maximum
	25–29	130	157	185
	30–34	126	153	180
	35–39	123	149	175
	40–44	119	145	170
	45–49	116	140	165
	50–54	112	136	160
	55–59	109	132	155
	60–64	105	128	150
	65 +	102	123	145
Men	**Age**	**Minimum**	**Optimum**	**Maximum**
	25–29	137	166	195
	30–34	133	162	190
	35–39	130	157	185
	40–44	126	153	180
	45–49	123	149	175
	50–54	119	145	170
	55–59	116	140	165
	60–64	112	136	160
	65 +	109	132	155

POOL WARM-UP

Enter the pool and begin bouncing or jogging easily for several minutes to increase slowly the demand placed on your heart. After this warm-up, choose exercise 1 or 2 or 3, any of which can be your complete aerobic workout for the day. Or choose the water circuit exercises, 4 through 8. If you desire increased aerobic benefits, and are already well-conditioned, select your basic aerobic exercise (1, 2, or 3), then follow it with the aerobic water circuit.

Exercise 1 SUSPENDED AEROBIC WATER RUNNING

You will need a flotation belt and a rope or elastic band for tether. Put on the flotation belt and turn it backward as in photo 1. Fasten one end of the tether around your waist and one end to a fixture at the side of the pool or to a dock in a lake, river, or bay. Suspended on the tether you need not worry about your footing or about running into others. You can close your eyes and concentrate on your running form.

Run for 20 minutes.

Running with companions can pull you to a harder workout than you might get alone. Take turns coaching and timing each other.

Photo 1

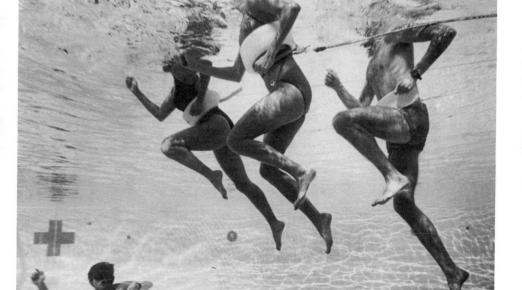

Exercise 2 AEROBIC WATER RUNNING

(Do this instead of exercise 1. Or do 1 **and** 2, each for 10 minutes.)

Run in chest-deep water back and forth across the pool, making each turn quickly enough to keep your heart rate up to target. At that speed your arm action should churn the water as in photo 2.

Exercise 3 BACKSTROKE ON TETHERS

If you can't swim but you **want** to swim as an aerobic exercise, try this assisted swimming device: the Greenberg Float Coat.

Put on the Float Coat. This will hold you above the water so you don't have to worry about sinking no matter how gently or vigorously you work. Attach the two tethers to a railing, ladder, or other fixture at the side of the pool. Lean back with your head at the surface of the water and begin kicking. Your legs will rise to the surface. Now begin alternating your arms in a backward circular motion (photo 3). As you perfect the backstroke you will be able to increase your speed and so raise your heart rate to your target zone. Over the weeks to come you will easily build your swim time to 10 minutes, then even-

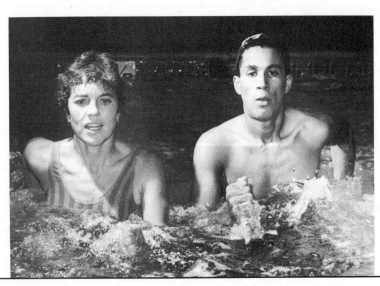

Photo 2

tually to 20 minutes. Until you've built up to 20 minutes of swimming, use this exercise in combination with exercise 1 or 2 to keep your heart rate in the target zone for the prescribed length of time.

If you are already a swimmer, start with a full 20-minute swim on the tethers, which keep you from bumping into people or having to turn at each end of the pool. Your attention can be completely focused on your strokes.

WATER CIRCUIT TRAINING

Each of these circuit exercises lasts 2 minutes, for a total of 10 minutes for one complete circuit. You must do the circuit twice in order to accumulate the 20 minutes necessary for an aerobic training effect.

At the end of your first circuit, take your pulse to monitor your working heart rate. Count the heartbeats for 6 seconds and add a zero to get your **working heart rate.** If you haven't been working hard enough on the first circuit, your heart rate may be 20 or 30 beats below your target zone. If you're working too hard, you may have overshot your target zone, which will make doing your second circuit difficult. As soon as you've

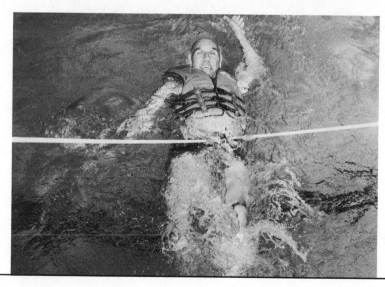

Photo 3

determined your working heart rate, begin your second circuit, modifying your rate of work: If your working heart rate is too slow, speed up. If it is too fast, slow down.

(Notice that you have used 6 seconds instead of 30 seconds as on page 69 for taking your heart rate. That's because your heart rate would drop quickly during the 30 seconds of standing still. **You must keep moving in this aerobic circuit.**)

Exercise 4 KICKBOARD—CIRCUIT, STATION 1

Circuit training can be done aerobically by working at each exercise hard enough to elevate your heart rate to target and then by moving swiftly to the next exercise station.

Exercises 4 through 8 are five stations of a pool training

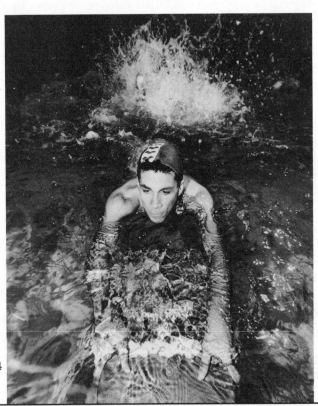

Photo 4

circuit. Begin with laps of flutter kicking, using a kickboard as in photo 4. Do this simple exercise to initiate a gradual increase in your working heart rate. Flutter kick for 2 minutes, stopping in the shallow end of the pool.

Exercise 5 MOVING FROG JUMPS—CIRCUIT, STATION 2

Leave your board at the shallow end of the pool. Bouncing on both feet, jump high and pull both knees toward your chest. Use your arms to initiate each jump and to gain extra height. Photo 5 shows the position at the top of a jump. This exercise takes a lot of effort, as you can see by the water's disturbance. Frog jump across your pool for 1 minute. Continue crossing and recrossing the pool with backward frog jumps for 1 minute.

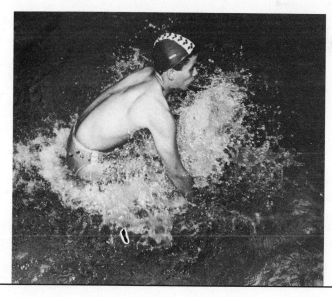

Photo 5

Exercise 6 LADDER ARM PRESS—CIRCUIT, STATION 3

Your legs are now tired from kicking and jumping; your arms are ready to work. Move quickly to the ladder.

Brace your feet against the pool wall or the bottom of the pool, depending on the depth of the water. Hold the ladder tightly with both hands. Pull inward (photo 6), then push out. Pull and push in rapid succession. Choose a speed and effort level that you can maintain for at least 2 minutes before moving back to the shallow end of the pool. Keep your body straight. Do not bend at the waist or hips.

Photo 6

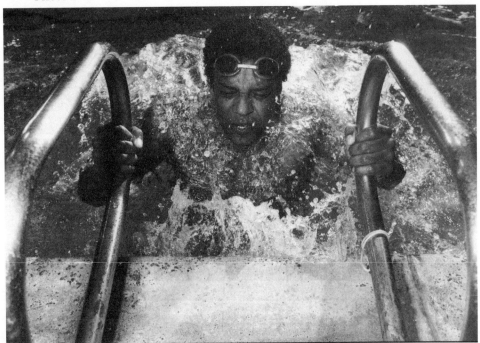

Exercise 7 ONE-LEGGED FROG JUMPS—CIRCUIT, STATION 4

Bounce on your right leg and hold your left knee bent in front of you as in photo 7. The left knee remains in this position throughout the exercise. Your arms can be out to your sides for balance. Now push off hard with your right leg and lift your right knee up to meet your left knee. Then drop your right foot and prepare for another push-off. Continue for 1 minute, then change legs. Jump on your left foot with your right knee held stationary in front of you. Repeat the exercise for 1 minute, then move quickly to station 5.

Photo 7

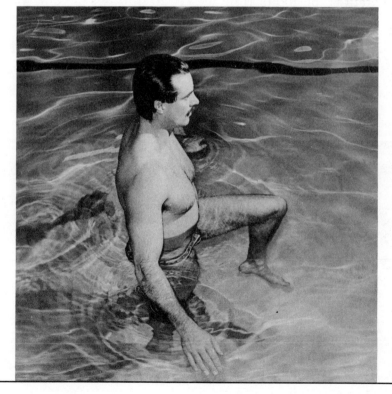

Exercise 8 AEROBIC SPORTS SKILLS—CIRCUIT, STATION 5

From your own favorite sport, choose a skill that adapts to the pool. Repeat the skill vigorously and continuously for 2 minutes. The weight lifter in photo 8 cleans and jerks an Olympic barbell repeatedly for 2 minutes.

Repeat the entire circuit.

THE ULTIMATE WORKOUT

If you've easily completed all of this program without seriously challenging your capacities, try this specific combination of programs designed for the high intensity competitive athlete:

Start with exercises 1 through 11 in the Basic Water Workout. Then, to keep your heart rate elevated for an extended period of time, insert 20 minutes of your Water Aerobic exercise (1, 2, or 3), followed by two loops of Water Circuit Training. Then return to the Basic Water Workout, continuing with exercises 12 through 20, which work all the major muscle groups of the body. Finally, add to this several sets of your sport-specific exercise (Chapter 7), then warm down with the Water Stretch.

Photo 8

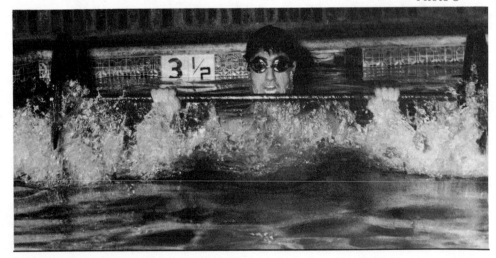

WATER AEROBICS WORKOUT

POOL WARM-UP
1. SUSPENDED AEROBIC WATER RUNNING 20 minutes*

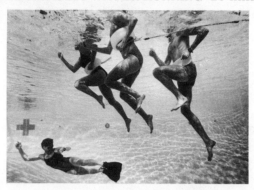

2. AEROBIC WATER RUNNING 20 minutes*
* OR: 10 minutes of #1 plus 10 minutes of # 2

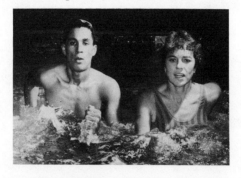

3. BACKSTROKE ON TETHERS 10 to 20 minutes

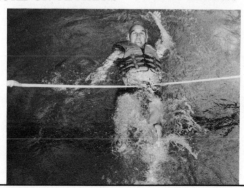

continued on page 82

WATER AEROBICS WORKOUT continued

WATER CIRCUIT TRAINING

4. *KICKBOARD FORWARD*
   2 minutes

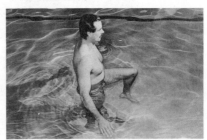

5. *MOVING FROG JUMPS*
   2 minutes

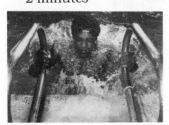

6. *LADDER ARM PRESS*
   2 minutes

7. *ONE-LEGGED FROG JUMPS*
   2 minutes

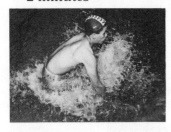

8. *AEROBIC SPORTS DRILLS*
   2 minutes

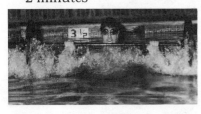

Monitor heart rate.
Repeat circuit exercises 4 through 8

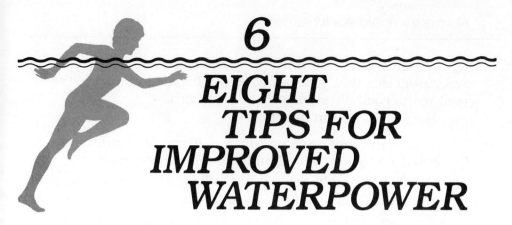

6

EIGHT TIPS FOR IMPROVED WATERPOWER

After several weeks on any fitness program, you may feel your initial euphoria begin to wear off. Doubts and problems may cause you to skip your workout once, then again, and eventually to give up your fitness program altogether, even though you are noticing beneficial results.

In the following sections you will find suggestions that will help you overcome 90 percent of your excuses for wanting to stay home instead of leaving for the pool. Concentrate on these tips before your next water workout.

1. KEEP YOUR GOALS FIRMLY IN MIND

When you think about what you want to accomplish in your water training, be as specific as you can. You may even want to write these goals down and keep them in a prominent place—on your nightstand, next to the phone, on the refrigerator door. Goal setting will be the crucial element of sticking to a water exercise program. Without daily, monthly, and lifetime goals you will be tempted to work out only occasionally, or not at all if pressed for time and energy.

Lifetime goals are universally the same as for other fitness programs that you may have participated in during the past years: good physical and mental health.

Monthly goals can be set by:

- Your bathroom scale and mirror if you are working toward losing weight and building muscle definition
- Your racquetball, tennis, basketball, or other scores if you aim for improvement in your sport
- Your lowered resting heart rate if you are seeking improved cardiovascular fitness
- The comparative ease with which your mind and body handle the demands of pregnancy
- The renewal and recuperation of your body if you have been ill or injured

As you think about your goals, you begin building the necessary willpower to accomplish them. Begin seeing your future body now. Imagine the feeling of doubled strength and power. Don't wait for some distant unknown time when you will have **arrived** at those goals; rather, begin enjoying the process you are going through **now.** You are moving toward your goal and you should feel good about each forward step you take.

Fitness sets the tone for much of your life. Your fitness level affects your moods, your relationships, the way you sleep, eat, work, and play. Fitness is not a luxury—it is the key to a satisfying life.

2. ESTABLISH A WORKOUT SCHEDULE

We are creatures of habit. Once water workouts have become a habit in your life, you will be less likely to skip a session. To make your workouts a habit, you must schedule them as a regular part of your day, not as an afterthought.

Carefully think through your time commitments and the

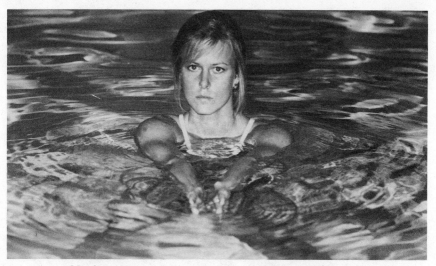

*Marlene Harmon has an appointment in 30 minutes
so she does only arm exercises and Water Stretch.*

physical logistics of getting to the pool. Give yourself enough
time. If you try to squeeze only a few minutes from your busy
day to hurry through a few fast exercises, you'll no doubt find
that you are spending more time and energy watching the
clock than thinking about your workout. Choose a suitable
time that meets these criteria:

- You will not be unduly rushed
- The pool will have room for you to work out
- You will not have eaten a meal within 2 to 3 hours
- The chance that family, work, or other commitments will
interrupt you is unlikely.

Do Waterpower Workouts three or more times a week if
they are your only major form of exercise. If you are training
regularly in another activity—aerobic dance, bicycling, running, playing basketball—use the water as your secondary

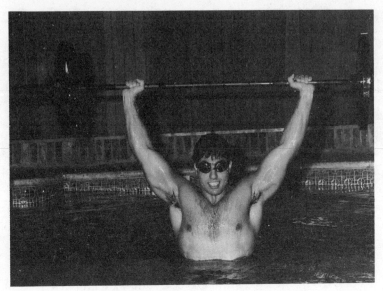

This athlete increases his weight-lifting
capacity through water training.

training program at least twice a week. Serious athletes can use water exercises daily if they wish. Most visit the pool *after* their regular sport workout in order to take the "edge" off their sore muscles. Others come to the pool *instead* of their regular workout if they have a slight injury, or if they feel they are reaching the critical area of potential injury due to over-training.

3. FIND A TRAINING PARTNER OR A WATER EXERCISE CLASS

A training partner in any sport can be vital to motivation. The companionship of someone with the same goals of improvement and persistence will stimulate you to stay with the daily routine. With someone alongside you to evaluate your performance, you move more quickly and steadily toward your goals. But remember: **Never wait for your training partner!** If your partner can't make it to a workout, be prepared to go alone. Don't let your partner determine **your** progress.

Some days your motivational level may be low. You might be tempted to skip your water workout unless you know that other people are waiting for you at the pool. Even on an "off" day, you'll bounce as high, jump as far, and work as hard as those around you in a group class.

If you can't find an existing water exercise program near you, discuss such a class with your friends. If you find enough interest, approach the director of your local health club or "Y." Offer to bring in a ready-made class if they will supply an instructor. If you feel qualified to teach the class, suggest that.

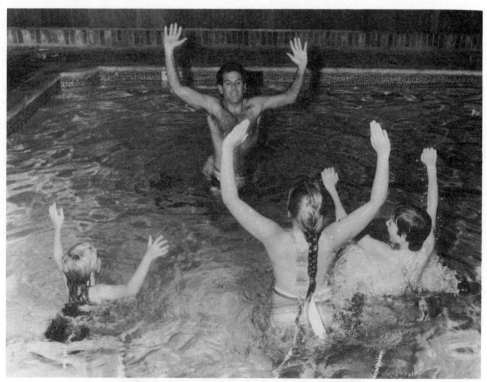

*Dr. Mike Greenberg shows young children that
Waterpower works for all ages.*

4. CONCENTRATE

Because you are immersing yourself in an unusual and soothing environment, your mental focus changes. But this new environment can also tend to make you dreamy; you can easily lose sight of your goals for that day's workout.

Concentration stems from believing in the importance of your goals. Remind yourself of those goals as you are changing into your bathing suit.

Think positively. Prefeel the sensations you like best during your water workout; the immediate pleasure of entering the water; the sense of power that spreads through your

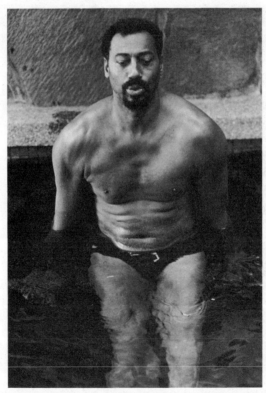

Wilt Chamberlain improves his water therapy with concentration.

thighs as you jump your highest; the satisfaction you feel after the hardest sprint interval. Think ahead to the most difficult part of your training program. Visualize yourself going through those exercises effortlessly. When you reach that part of your program, mentally return to your vision and try to match it. If you begin to tire, try to work through the fatigue with mental toughness. Often you will get a wave of renewed strength if you're willing to push through that first barrier.

5. IGNORE CURIOUS ONLOOKERS

The first time you do your water workout in a new pool, you may see several people watching your unique exercises. Don't let their stares stop you. Keep your attention focused on your exercises, your form, and your developing strength. Do not look around and become involved with other people in the pool, kids playing, or hot dog divers. Concentrate on your workout and keep moving. Don't allow conversations to interrupt your workout. If curious onlookers ask you about your exercises, tell them you will explain **after** you have finished.

6. ESTABLISH YOUR WORKOUT SPACE IN THE POOL

Before you enter the water, note the movement patterns that have already been established by those training in the pool. Then choose an area of the pool for your workout that will least interfere. Once you're in the water, immediately establish your own work space. Do several arm swings and leg swings to show those around you the size of your work space. Try to stay within the space you first map out for yourself, especially if the pool is busy. Then get to work and keep your attention on your own workout. Others will respect your space if you take your work seriously.

7. NOTICE SIDE BENEFITS

While you warm down, take time to notice any side benefits you may be receiving while water training.

Because water is a natural tranquilizer you may be feeling more calm than usual. You may be sleeping better. You may experience improved digestion and fewer headaches after you have established a habit of working out in water.

Perhaps you've noticed that the water soothes away the aches and pains that often accompany the first day of menstrual flow. Even if you don't feel 100 percent, you can do your workout. Start slowly and let your body dictate the effort level for the day's workout. If you feel a bit weak or tired when you begin, do the first few exercises gently. You may be pleasantly surprised to feel your strength building during the session. Even if you start your water workout with menstrual cramps, you'll find that moving slowly and gently through all the exercises will make you feel better overall.

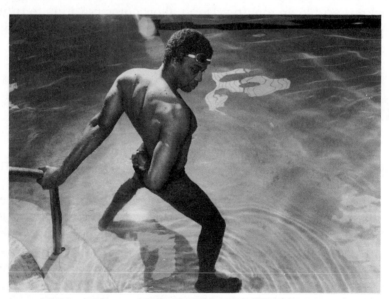

Bernie Casey savors his favorite shoulder stretch

Perhaps you spent years wishing for a sport that did not make you feel awkward. Waterpower programs may be the first activity in which you feel truly athletic. Take that new-found confidence away from the pool with you.

You may have just learned that the serious intent you bring to a workout can be applied to other aspects of your life with the same successful results. As soon as you tap into that inner power available to you in workouts, you will quickly learn to channel it into all parts of your life.

8. HAVE FUN

Find a favorite stretch or exercise that you particularly enjoy, then savor it.

Smile, laugh, even sing if you feel the urge as water cheers you and brings out your best.

Take a minute after your workout to relax and enjoy the soothing water. If you can swim, float for a minute or so. If not, hold on to the side of the pool, close your eyes, and let the water rock you for a few moments.

Congratulate yourself on work well done.

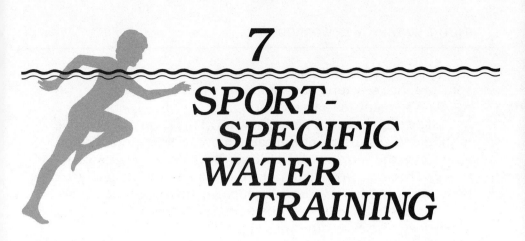

7
SPORT-
SPECIFIC
WATER
TRAINING

Human movement patterns cannot be repeated exactly. Chris Evert's ground strokes from the baseline, however similar they may look during a 2-hour tennis match on TV, are never identical. Neither are the golf drives of Arnold Palmer, the strides of Joan Benoit in a marathon, the compulsory figures of a skater, nor the strokes of an ultradistance swimmer from England to France to England. No two human movements can ever be identical.

Nonetheless, athletes train daily to acquire these grooved moves, always hoping to find that one "sweet spot," then repeat it and repeat it, trying to make it their **only** spot. Think, for example about your own foul shots in basketball. You've probably worked very hard on a ritual so that each time you release the ball you have made the same moves beforehand: You've bounced the ball three times. You've set your feet precisely on the line. You've taken a deep breath. You've shut out all thought but the image of a swish as you bend your knees, lift your arms, and release. Yet during this entire process your body is combining and recombining each neural impulse into millions of different patterns. You're finding the grooves, all right. They're sweet spots. And you're always trying to refind them during your practice drills.

But such drills can become tedious and flat, no matter

what your level of skill, and tedium can lead to cutting short your practice sessions or to skipping them altogether.

You're ready for a fresh setting.

Try drilling at your sport in water. There you can practice with added zest many of the same moves you've practiced on land, only the moves will be slower because of water's resistance. These extra seconds per move allow you to feel your body parts in "freeze frame," which in turn gives you more time for feedback to correct the motions. Water drill gives you a new focus for assessing your skills.

Many of the exercises to follow are sport-specific skill drills. As you practice the ones pertinent to your sport, try to simulate as closely as possible the moves you ordinarily make on land. For example, when you are cross-country skiing in water (photo 6), maximize the exercise benefits by simulating the stride length and weight transfer you would actually use on snow.

Other of the exercises in this chapter are designed to build strength in the primary muscle groups needed for specific sports. Because increasing your strength automatically improves your skills, incorporating strength exercises into your water workout will improve your athletic performance. Many world-class athletes who have reached the upper level of their capacity to handle strength workouts on land are moving into water for at least one strength workout per week. In this way they can actually increase their number of sets and reps while preventing stress injuries that might occur if they tried to do the additional strength work on land. You can train like these Olympic and professional athletes by taking your sport into the pool.

BASEBALL

SKILL DRILL

Exercise 1 PRACTICE BASEBALL SWING

With an old baseball bat, take practice swings in a pool. Try bunting, then try switch-hitting.

STRENGTH EXERCISE

Exercise 2 WATER MEDICINE BALL

Latissimus dorsi, abdominal obliques, pectorals, quadratus lumborum

Stand in chest-deep water with your feet comfortably apart for balance. Hold a large ball with both hands, arms straight out to the left as Bart Gallagher does in photo 2A. Kim Gallagher shows how the exercise can be done without a ball. Keeping your arms straight, start a semicircular movement by pushing the ball down through the water. Guide the ball across the front of your body. The ball will surface to the right of your body (photo 2B). Move the ball back through that same semicircle in the opposite direction. Without the ball, Kim follows the same movement sequence using only her flat hand, fingers together. This exercise, as well as others you

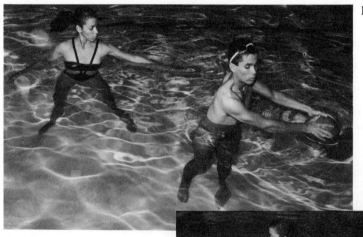

Photo 2A

Photo 2B

continued on page 96

may create with the water medicine ball, will strengthen your chest, shoulders, and back for baseball, basketball, golf, bowling, and other sports. Any large ball is difficult to submerge when fully inflated. The more difficult, the more force you must exert.

BASKETBALL

SKILL DRILL

Exercise 3 JUMP SHOT WITH DRAG SUIT

Find a training partner and an old basketball to take to the pool. Perform your normal jump shot, jumping as high as you can each time (photo 3). The Arena drag suit Bernie Casey wears increases the workload as he jumps. Shoot toward your partner. When the ball is returned, jump high and shoot again. Repeat 25 times.

If a sore knee or ankle won't permit jumping on land, you can retain your timing and jumping ability with this exercise.

(You might be able to persuade your pool director to install a backboard.)

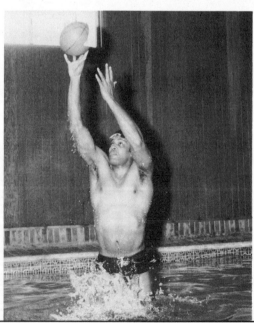

Photo 3

SKILL DRILL

Exercise 4 BLOCK SHOT WITH DRAG SUIT

WORKING PARTNER: Your training partner holds the ball and motions you forward, or left, or right, or backward. As soon as you see the exaggerated motion, jump in that direction as though blocking a shot. The drag suit will provide extra water resistance (photo 4).

COACHING PARTNER: Move quickly, thrusting the ball either front, back, left, or right with an exaggerated motion. Hold that position while your partner reacts. Remember that movement is slower in water than on land. Vary your signals so that a pattern doesn't emerge. In this way, your partner will have a true reaction/movement exercise.

This same exercise can be done without a partner, as in shadow boxing. This added resistance will overload the muscles that propel you through the water. Consequently, those muscles will become stronger.

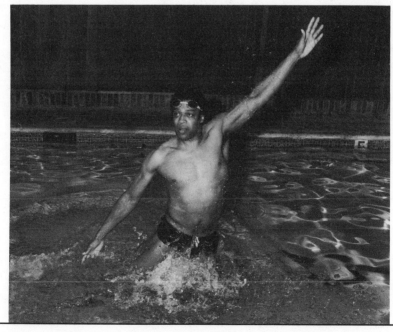

Photo 4

CYCLING

STRENGTH EXERCISE

Exercise 5 PARTNER LEG PRESS
Quadriceps, abdominals, feet flexors, and extensors

WORKING PARTNER: Brace yourself with your back to the side of the pool. Bend your knees to your chest as in photo 5A. Push forcefully against your partner, extending your legs to position 5B. Pull and push 25 times for added strength in cycling, running, and jumping.

COACHING PARTNER: Grasp your partner's ankles firmly and hold them tightly against your shoulders or upper chest. Stand with one foot a full stride in front of the other for lever-

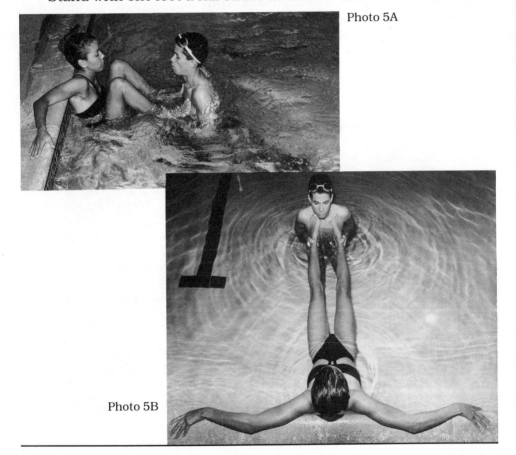

Photo 5A

Photo 5B

age. As your partner pushes against you, lean forward for resistance. Lean backward as your partner begins to pull. Breathe out each time the water begins to wash over you. Offer more or less resistance according to your partner's wishes.

CROSS-COUNTRY SKIING

SKILL DRILL

Exercise 6 STRIDE PRACTICE

Slide your feet along the bottom of the pool and swing your arms as though cross-country skiing (photo 6). The harder you work, the more the water will offer counterforce. Use the clock to time your training session inasmuch as you can't measure your distance. Add weight gloves to build poling power. Add ankle weights when you want to work your legs harder.

Photo 6

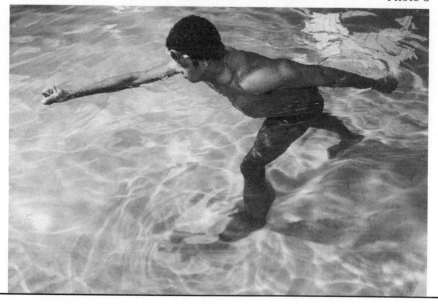

DISCUS

SKILL DRILL

Exercise 7 KEY POSITION PRACTICE

A key position in throwing the discus is driving across the circle, then dropping low enough so that the foreleg is nearly parallel to the ground. Although gold medalist Mac Wilkins can assume and hold this difficult position on land (photo 7), many discus throwers cannot.

Match Mac's position in the water. The support of the water allows you to assume his position and learn the "feel" of it. In water, carefully duplicate the correct bend of the legs and proper height of the hips as you drive through this critical position. Mac says he can do more repetitions in water than he can on land. Also, he reports that his range of motion is dramatically increased in water.

Use this same concept of isolating and learning a key body position for any sport that requires complex yet precise motor skills, such as gymnastics, javelin throwing, figure skating, or shot putting.

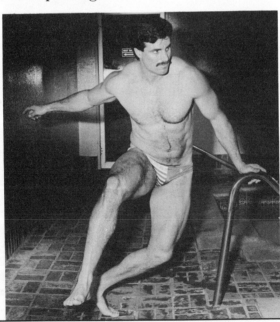

Photo 7

SKILL DRILL

Exercise 8 ROTATION PRACTICE

Do the entire discus rotation in the pool. Although speed will be lost due to water resistance, accuracy of precise movements is increased. (See photos 8A and 8B.)

Photo 8A

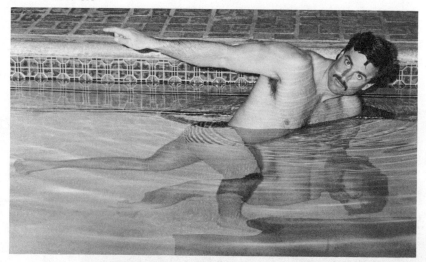

Photo 8B

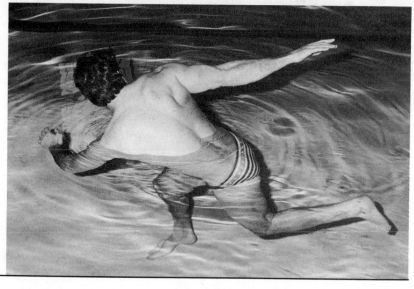

FOOTBALL/RUGBY

SKILL DRILL

Exercise 9 CATCH

Practice the hand-eye coordination of catching the football while you're in the pool. You must work harder than you would on land to move quickly through the dense water to reach the ball (photo 9). Sharpen your concentration so that you don't drop the slippery football once you've caught it. This exercise is good mental and physical practice.

Photo 9

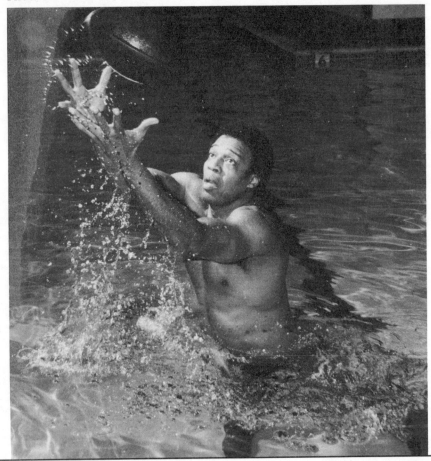

SKILL DRILL

Exercise 10 RUN, NO FUMBLE

Tuck the football into your chest as Bernie does in photo 10. Run back and forth across the pool 10 times, maintaining a firm grip on the ball. For variety, you can mix exercises 9 and 10. First catch the ball, then run across the pool without fumbling.

Photo 10

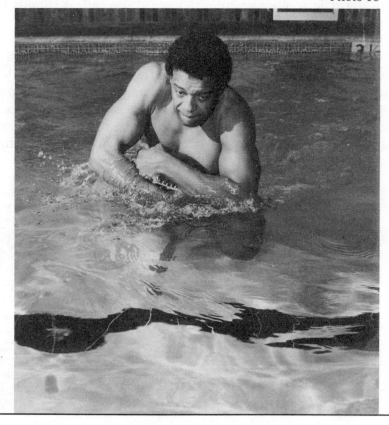

GOLF

SKILL DRILL

Exercise 11 PRACTICE GOLF SWING

Take an old iron or wooden club into the pool with you and practice your golf swing. Use the slowed-down motion to evaluate your arm, wrist, and hip action.

STRENGTH EXERCISE

Exercise 12 PARTNER ARM PRESS

Lats, deltoids, triceps, biceps, pecs, wrist flexors, and extensors

WORKING PARTNER: Firmly grip a ladder, railing, or pool gutter with both hands. Bring your legs to the surface behind you. Bend your elbows and pull toward the railing (photo 12). Keep both knees and your back straight as you extend your elbows and push back against your partner.

COACHING PARTNER: Hold your partner's feet tightly against your stomach or chest. As the working partner pulls in, lean back to offer resistance against the movement. As your partner pushes out, lean forward. Give more or less resistance as your partner requests. If you experience difficulty in maintaining a grip on your partner's ankles, tuck the feet under your arms and squeeze.

Photo 12

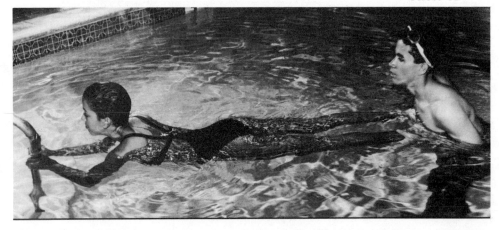

MARTIAL ARTS

STRENGTH EXERCISE

Exercise 13 TREE POSE

Deltoids, trapezius, gluteals, quads, abdominals

Stand on your left foot while you focus your gaze steadily on a spot about eye level. Place your right foot as high on your left inner thigh as possible. Raise both arms above you, holding a kickboard or other object overhead. (See photo 13). Tuck your tailbone down in order to prevent standing swayback. Hold this position while you breathe deeply five times. Repeat on the right foot.

Although balancing seems easier in the water than on land, you must keep your gaze steady and your concentration firm. These qualities will transfer to your discipline in the martial arts.

If you have any difficulty with this exercise, start by holding on to the side of the pool and gradually move away.

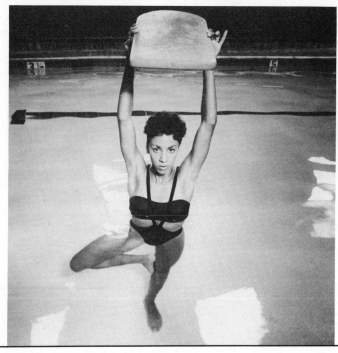

Photo 13

RACKET SPORTS

SKILL DRILL

Exercise 14 PRACTICE RACKET SWING

Choose your oldest racket to take into the water. Practice walking through the swinging motion of each of your strokes (photo 14). Because the water slows you down, you have the opportunity to feel each segment of your stroke and work on any weak or awkward spot. Good strokes are the heart of the game. If you want to play better, you must improve them.

Change hands and work the other side of the body to prevent body imbalances that often come from unilateral sports.

Photo 14

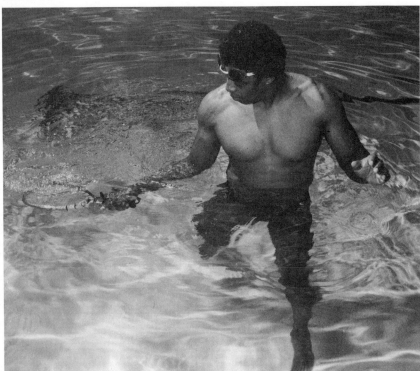

STRENGTH EXERCISE

Exercise 15 TIDAL WAVE

Pecs, biceps, triceps, lats, wrist flexors

In chest-deep water, tightly hold a ladder, railing, or gutter with both hands. Elbows are straight (photo 15A). Keep the body straight as you bend your elbows and pull inward (photo 15B). As you speed up the push-pull movement, the force required will increase. Do 15 push-pull cycles at top speed. Recover. Repeat for grip and chest strength in racket sports, golf, and holding ski poles.

Photo 15A

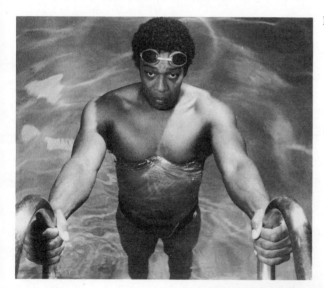

Photo 15B

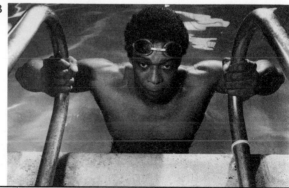

RUNNING

SKILL DRILL

Exercise 16 SPRINTING ON TETHER

WORKING PARTNER: Sprint in place in chest-deep water, pulling against an elastic tether attached to the side of the pool (photo 16). The tether allows you to lean forward into proper sprinting position. Run your interval workout based on times that seek to duplicate distances. For example, run five 45 second sprints to approximate five 300 meter sprints.

COACHING PARTNER: Call out times (as in split times) every 15 seconds.

Variation—Fartlek

WORKING PARTNER: Now take off the tether to prepare for fartlek (speed play). Your coach will use imagination to link a variety of running speeds. For example, your coach will call for you to sprint across the pool at top speed, driving your arms as hard as your legs, then turn and run slowly back, then turn, sprint, jog, turn, two sprint laps, and so on.

COACHING PARTNER: Watch your athlete's face and breathing for signs of fatigue. Provide a hard workout but also allow recovery time between sprint phases.

Runners who are injured often use these exercises in the water to retain their fitness while leg injuries heal.

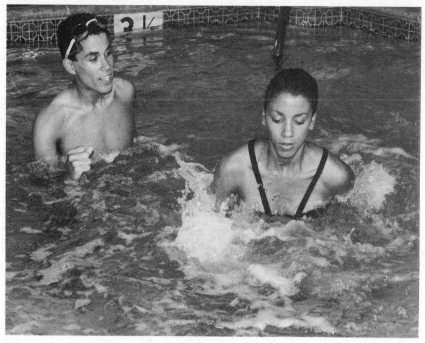

Photo 16

SOCCER

SKILL DRILL

Exercise 17 PRACTICE KICK

Without a ball, work on your football, rugby, and soccer kicks in waist-deep water, focusing primarily on form. The water will slow down the movement and allow you to "feel" each phase of the kick.

Emphasize the point of contact and the follow-through. Practice with both feet, spending more time on the weaker foot.

STRENGTH EXERCISE

Exercise 18 JUMP ON COMMAND

Abdominals, abdominal obliques, quads, hamstrings, gastrocs

WORKING PARTNER: Begin jumping in place on both feet. Arms are relaxed at your sides. By not using your arms, you must initiate the movement with the muscles of the abdomen and trunk—muscles that must be highly developed in proficient soccer, volleyball, football, and basketball players. Concentrate on reacting instantly to the sound of your partner's voice. As Bart yells "Front, back, left, right," Kim jumps immediately in that direction (photo 18).

COACHING PARTNER: Vary your calls so your partner can't predict your pattern. In this way, every command causes an instant decision and reaction before the quick movement.

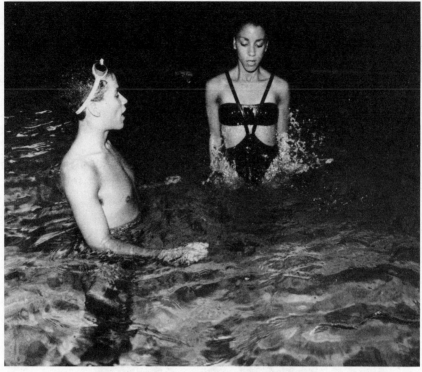

Photo 18

VOLLEYBALL

SKILL DRILL

Exercise 19 BLOCK WITH DRAG SUIT

WORKING PARTNER: React quickly to each spiked ball that is hit toward you. Jump high (photo 19), blocking the ball into the water. Watch the ball until you've made contact with it. Toss the ball back to your partner and prepare for the next block.

COACHING PARTNER: Spike an old volleyball toward your partner. Vary the speed of your hits. Your partner will time his or her jump and block accordingly.

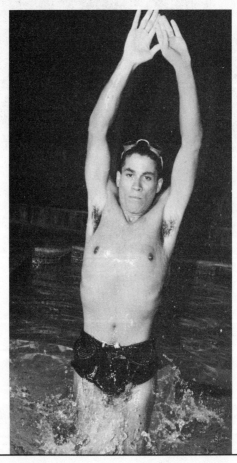

Photo 19

CUSTOMIZE YOUR PROGRAM

The photos in this chapter should trigger ideas for designing your own sport-specific water program. Here are several examples:

- You're a triathlete. Think up a way to ride your oldest bike on a stationary platform in neck-deep water.
- You're a soccer coach. Take the entire team to an occasional kicking drill in water (see exercise 17). Devise also a heading drill.
- You're coaching your son or daughter. Analyze the developing skills in the tension-free atmosphere of a pool.
- You're a long jumper who hasn't quite mastered the in-flight leg movements of the jump. Have your coach watch you work at it in chest-deep water.
- You're a gymnast with a sprained ankle who swims and water runs to maintain conditioning. Before you leave the pool, practice the dance portions of your free exercise routine in chest-deep water.

Finally, try adding more exercises from this chapter to your sport-specific program. Use the following chart for suggestions.

SPORT-SPECIFIC WATER TRAINING

Sport		
Archery	Exercise 2	Water Medicine Ball
Baseball	Exercise 1	Practice Baseball Swing
	Exercise 2	Water Medicine Ball
	Exercise 15	Tidal Wave
Basketball	Exercise 2	Water Medicine Ball
	Exercise 3	Jump Shot
	Exercise 4	Block Shot
	Exercise 5	Partner Leg Press
	Exercise 15	Tidal Wave
	Exercise 18	Jump on Command

continued on page 114

SPORT-SPECIFIC WATER TRAINING continued

Sport

Bowling	Exercise 2	Water Medicine Ball
	Exercise 5	Partner Leg Press
	Exercise 15	Tidal Wave
Cycling	Exercise 5	Partner Leg Press
	Exercise 16	Sprinting/Fartlek
Cross-Country Skiing	Exercise 5	Partner Leg Press
	Exercise 6	Stride Practice
	Exercise 15	Tidal Wave
Discus	Exercise 7	Key Position Practice
	Exercise 8	Rotation Practice
Football/Rugby	Exercise 9	Catch
	Exercise 10	Run, No Fumble
	Exercise 17	Practice Kick
	Exercise 18	Jump on Command
Golf	Exercise 2	Water Medicine Ball
	Exercise 11	Practice Swing
	Exercise 12	Partner Arm Press
	Exercise 15	Tidal Wave
Martial Arts	Exercise 5	Partner Leg Press
	Exercise 12	Partner Arm Press
	Exercise 13	Tree Pose
Racket Sports	Exercise 2	Water Medicine Ball
	Exercise 5	Partner Leg Press
	Exercise 14	Practice Racket Swing
	Exercise 15	Tidal Wave
Running	Exercise 5	Partner Leg Press
	Exercise 16	Sprinting/Fartlek
Soccer	Exercise 5	Partner Leg Press
	Exercise 16	Sprinting/Fartlek
	Exercise 17	Practice Kick
	Exercise 18	Jump on Command
Volleyball	Exercise 12	Partner Arm Press
	Exercise 18	Jump on Command
	Exercise 19	Volleyball Block

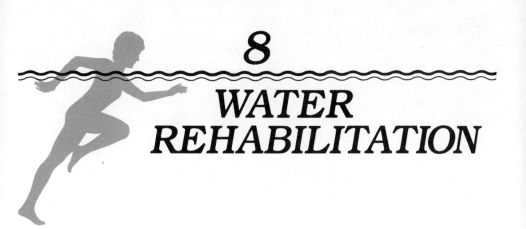

8

WATER REHABILITATION

August 1983: Helsinki, Finland: Olympic Stadium

Cuba's double gold medalist (1976), Alberto Juantoreno, crossed the finish line of an 800 meter heat on his way to a probable gold medal at the first World Athletic Championships. But as he slowed, a Kenyan runner collided with Alberto, causing him to trip and land precariously on his right foot, then fall to the infield. He tore the lateral ligaments of his right ankle and broke his fifth metatarsal bone. Finnish surgeons immediately repaired the ligament damage and put a cast on Alberto's foot so the broken bone would be immobilized as it healed.

I visited my friend Alberto in his hospital room a few hours after surgery. His was the ultimate frustration of any athlete: His body was finely tuned, capable of winning, but his foot could never have left any starting line. He bravely predicted a fast comeback, and I encouraged him to use Cuba's warm waters as part of his rehabilitation program when the cast came off.

He did. Six months later I heard from him that a morning swim had become a regular part of his training routine.

In the past decade, the treatment of sports injuries has evolved into a sophisticated science. Injuries that were once disabling are being rehabilitated, allowing athletes to return quickly—dramatically—to competition.

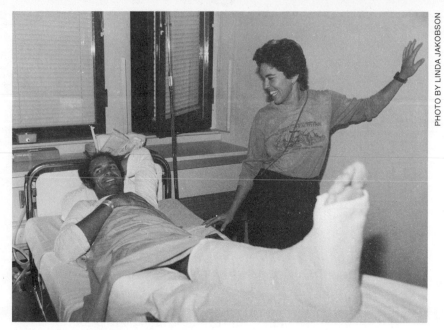

Lynda Huey visits Cuban Olympian Alberto Juantorena in Helsinki, advising on water's use in his rehabilitation program.

Water therapy is one of these "miracles" used in rehabilitating a whole range of sprains, strains, dislocations, and fractures. More specifically, exercising in water is becoming the standard treatment for injured athletes. Water accelerates healing by improving circulation to the injured body part so that it does not stiffen up and lose all motion. Water also protects (by supporting) the injured body part during exercise that would be stressful on land.

Use the water therapy described in this chapter to treat similar injuries, or to enhance your current rehabilitation program, keeping in mind these general principles:

• You never have to stop exercising. Work the uninjured body parts until you can tolerate movement in the injured area.

- Do gentle water therapy twice daily for the first two weeks. When you can handle longer sessions with increased resistance, do water therapy once a day.
- Do all water therapy exercises gently, smoothly, and with good biomechanics (form).
- If you encounter pain or discomfort, modify the exercise by moving more slowly through a narrower range of motion.
- Increase your workload—resistance, repetitions—**very gradually.**
- Work with your doctor, coach, or trainer so that you **know the reason** for doing a particular exercise.
- Before resuming your regular sport or activity, you should be pain-free and have reestablished full strength and range of motion in the injured part.

DISCOVERING WATER'S HEALING POWER

I depend on water whenever the slightest ache or pain makes me leery of an upcoming track workout. Instead of forcing that workout, I jump into the ocean or into a pool. I suspect that water has saved me from several potential injuries in recent years, injuries that were just waiting to happen because of overtraining. And when injury **does** strike (for even the best injury-prevention training program can't eliminate **all** injuries), I simply switch into my "swim gear" and continue training. Of all the benefits water training has brought to my life, the most important is that I have learned to save myself from the horrible depressions and loss of conditioning that injured athletes suffer.

Believe me; I learned the hard way:

The Amateur Athletic Union National Championships were two weeks away in June 1968. I'd sprinted well for San Jose State University during the collegiate season and had run a qualifying time for the 1968 Olympic Trials 100 meters.

I was far from a favorite to make the Mexico City Olympic team, but I had a shot at it if I trained longer and harder than I ever had before.

Tommie Smith, who would win gold in Mexico, took practice starts with me one cloudy afternoon before the Nationals. I struggled to stay with him out of the blocks, but in such fast company I strained too hard. The next morning I woke up with a painful Achilles' tendon, which kept me from training for two solid weeks. Thus I lost my conditioning and with it my long shot at the Olympics. I hadn't learned yet that I could have trained in water to avoid losing my conditioning while my Achilles healed.

Years later, in 1974, I was the coach of an Oberlin College basketball team. Because women's athletic teams in those days weren't provided with trainers, it was my job to oversee the fitness of my players. When my starting guard sprained her ankle early in the season, I iced the ankle, taped it, then put her on crutches. She played no more games that season only because I hadn't yet learned how to speed the recovery of an injury with water therapy, nor had I learned that water exercise could keep an injured athlete in shape for her return to competition.

It took an accident in 1976 in Beijing, China, to open my eyes to water's healing power.

Washington Redskin George Starke and I were in the airport, running to catch up with our sports delegation which had just completed a tour of China. I took a wrong step and turned my left foot. I couldn't ice it until we landed in Tokyo. Two days later, in Honolulu, I began to suspect that my foot was broken. George thought so too, but each day he urged me to swim with him in the ocean. The Redskins used water therapy on injured players at that time, and George reasoned that the ocean was natural water therapy, with its undulating motion and massaging effects.

Back home in Los Angeles a heavy cast on my left leg

severely limited my activity. When the cast was cut off, I was horrified to see a scrawny, atrophied ankle and calf. I soaked it daily in hot baths, massaging it to force out the stiffness, to bring new blood for speeding recovery. Then, because it hurt to walk, I took to the water. In a large pool I made myself walk without a limp, using the water's support as my crutch. I learned that no matter how disabled I was on land, I wasn't crippled in the water.

Earlier in my athletic career, whenever I was sidelined with injury, my months of inactivity dragged by with agonizing frustration. I would lose muscle tone, gain weight, and become cranky. But with Waterpower, it is possible to get a reasonable workout within days after an injury. Recently during an indoor track meet, I tore my lower right hamstring. Yet only 4 days later I was in the pool, inventing new exercises. I jumped on one leg, and worked both my arms through the water. While my hamstring healed, I was able to maintain cardiovascular fitness and muscle tone. Best of all, I satisfied my itch for movement and avoided depression. At first, I barely swung my injured leg through the water, but as the muscle became stronger, I could work more actively against the water's resistance. The harder I pushed, the more the water's counterforce. Sooner than I expected, I regained full use of my leg and at the same time reaffirmed my belief in water rehabilitation.

HOW WATER REHABILITATION WORKS FOR YOUR BODY

1. ELBOW

Wilt Chamberlain had elbow surgery in which his tricep tendon was reattached to the bone. His right arm was in a cast for 4 weeks. The day the cast was removed he found he had severely limited movement in that elbow joint. Over the next few weeks Wilt sped up healing and increased the range of motion in his elbow by using water rehabilitation exercises in his home hot tub.

continued on page 120

In photo 1A, Wilt sits in the Jacuzzi and bends his elbow to full flexion. His elbows stay straight out to the sides throughout this exercise. Slowly he begins to extend his arms out to the side as in photo 1B. By the time he reaches the position in photo 1C he has fully extended his injured elbow and slowly contracted his tricep muscle through its full range of motion. He repeated this exercise slowly, 10 times the first few sessions, working primarily on gaining flexibility in his elbow. Two weeks later he could do 30 repetitions of this exercise.

Photo 1A

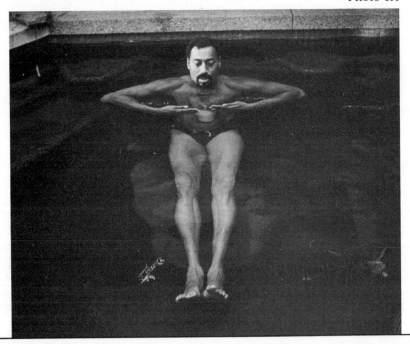

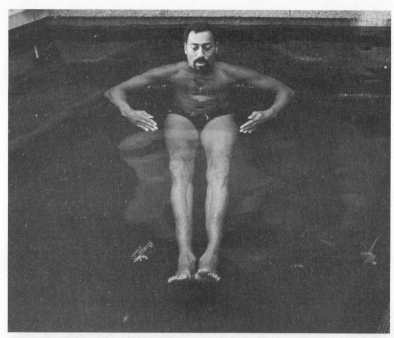

Photo 1B

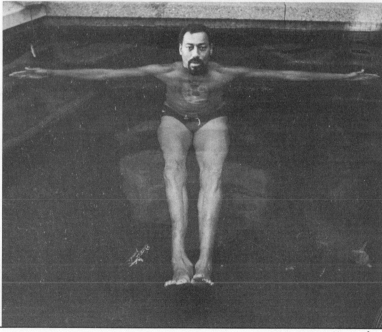

Photo 1C

continued on page 122

Once Wilt's elbow could tolerate heavier work, he did the semiweight-bearing movements in photos 1D and 1E. He placed both hands on a submerged ledge of his Jacuzzi and straightened his arms. His legs floated in front of him and his hips hung out over a deeper level of the Jacuzzi (1D). He bent both arms, lowering himself into the position in 1E. (Inadvertently he bent his right knee as he sought a balanced position.) Wilt then did 5, very slow up-down cycles of this backward dip and two weeks later had worked up to 30 reps.

Photo 1D

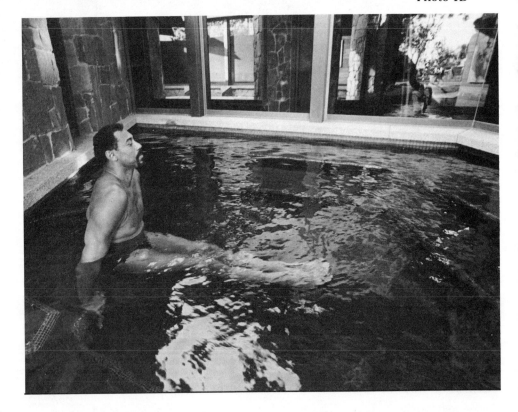

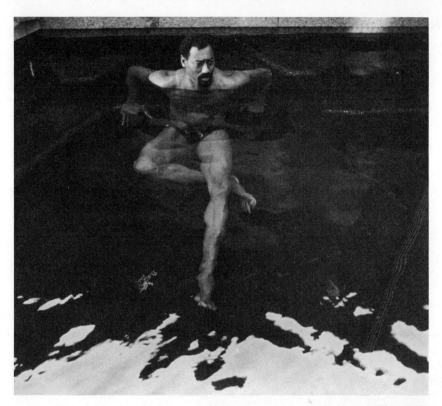

Photo 1E

2. SHOULDER

Here, in photo 2A, Dr. Mike Greenberg applies tape to an Olympic swimmer's separated shoulder. This functional taping limits her range of motion, thus keeping her arm from moving into a position that could further damage the joint. Now she's prepared to hold a 2-pound dumbbell and bend forward at the waist to describe small clockwise circles with her right arm (photo 2B). She will repeat with counterclockwise circles. Each day she will be able to do more reps and sets of this exercise, eventually using a 5-pound dumbbell.

Photo 2A

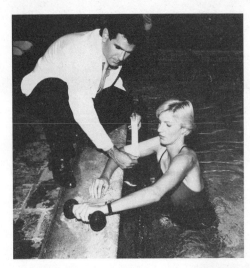

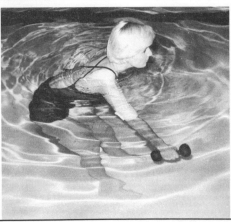

Photo 2B

3. CHEST

In photo 3A, Dr. Vicky Vodon's patient is a boxer who had occasional cramping in both pectoral muscles. He had been unable to find a stretch for relief until Dr. Vodon took him into shoulder-deep water and worked with him on the partner stretch pictured. (This photo was shot in shallow water in order to show clearly the involved body parts.) Later in the same water exercise program, Dr. Vodon's patient worked his arms and hands against a ball tethered to the bottom of the pool (3B). This target doesn't return a jolting shock, as would a punching bag.

Photo 3A

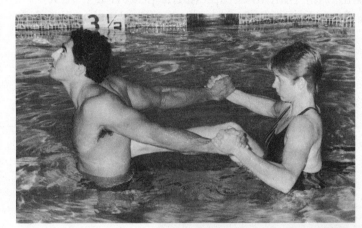

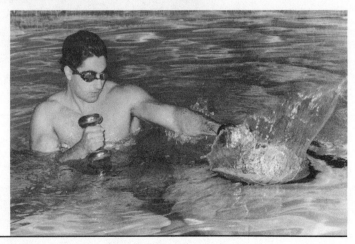

Photo 3B

4. LOWER BACK

Before Mac Wilkins began throwing the discus he was a golfer, tennis player, and football kicker and quarterback. All of these sports are unilateral activities; that is, they demand strength, speed, and power primarily from one side of the body. This one-sided body development over a lifetime had begun to cause problems: Mac has overdeveloped the right side of his body in comparison to his left side.

On and off for the past several years, Mac has been plagued by nerve pain in his right hip and in the right side of his lower back. When he performs a discus rotation, the pain makes it impossible for him to complete the powerful thrust that must come from his right leg just prior to releasing the disc. "Nothing helps but swimming with a flotation belt," he told his doctor.

The flotation belt lifts Mac's back, letting the tailbone rotate downward, relieving the pressure on his lower back. By swimming two or three times a week as in photo 4, Mac is able to alleviate his back problems within two weeks' time.

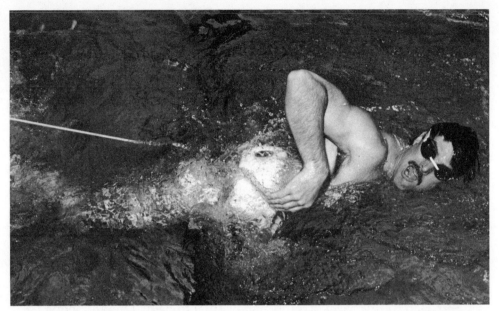

Photo 4

Mac has access to a large pool for swimming, but the tether (i.e., Perry-Band) can also be used in a small pool or in a cool-water Jacuzzi. The tether allows swimmers to concentrate on their strokes, for they need not concern themselves with bumping into other people or with making turns at the ends of the pool.

Here's how to use the elastic band and flotation device for the freestyle swimming stroke: (1) Strap a flotation device around your hips. Turn the strap to the back so that more flotation power will lift your hips once you start swimming; (2) pull the flotation belt down snugly around your hips; (3) attach one end of an elastic tether to your waist; (4) attach the other end to a ladder or railing on the side of the pool; (5) begin stroking. Goggles protect the eyes from chlorine; a mask and snorkel will free you from having to turn your head to breathe, thereby decreasing stress on your neck and upper back. All of your concentration can be given to your stroke.

5. *THIGH*

Torn hamstrings can go immediately into the water. Only two days after the injury (photo 5), Dr. Greenberg and the water support the leg as the knee is first bent, then straightened ever so slightly. These moves, as minimal as they are, help disperse the pooled blood collected around the site of the tear. Other than these cautious moves (if done on land they would cause pain), the knee is kept straight during the first week of water therapy. Functional taping supports the injured muscles, and in four days or so from the time of the injury these muscles can begin movement on their own. The wet tape is removed after each water rehabilitation session and new tape is applied.

As the hamstring heals and again can contract to bend the knee, it becomes important to regain full flexibility. Water stretching begins with the knee bent (as in exercise 4, Chapter 9) and gradually straightened over several weeks until a complete hamstring stretch has been achieved. The Acuscope and Myopulse, computerized electrotherapy, are used daily to decrease pain, reduce swelling, and speed healing. Used concurrently with water exercises, these instruments greatly accelerate healing time.

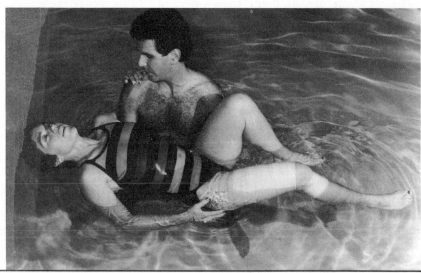

Photo 5

6. CALF

The masters' runner in photo 6 has shin splints, an inflammation of the connective tissue between the tibia (shinbone) and the adjacent muscles. (Shin splints are also common among aerobic dancers.) He hasn't been able to run on land because of the pain, but has just completed a 20-minute run with his feet barely touching the bottom of the pool: Shoulder-deep water has supported him. To complete this water therapy, Dr. Greenberg takes his patient through a series of resistance exercises. The runner flexes his feet as Dr. Greenberg resists, then the runner points his toes and Dr. Greenberg again resists. Together they work and resist **all** muscles of the calf and foot, performing movements in all possible directions.

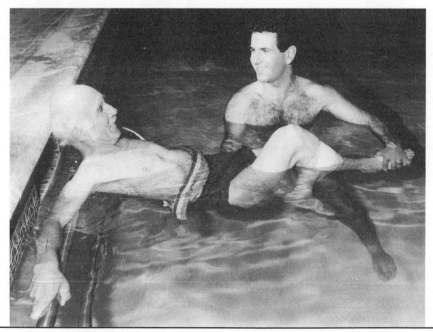

Photo 6

7. ANKLE

Photo 7 shows Candida Mobley rehabilitating her left ankle, which she sprained while teaching aerobic dancing. On land she can barely walk without limping, but in a flotation belt in the water she has little trouble with ankle flexions and extensions. (The tether is used only as a safety device in case she slips.) She lifts the heel of her left taped foot at the same time she lifts her right toes. Then she rocks both feet to the opposite positions, right heel up and left toes up. She repeats this exercise heel-toe, heel-toe, for 3 to 5 minutes in order to strengthen the muscles of her calf and foot and to regain ankle flexibility.

Photo 7

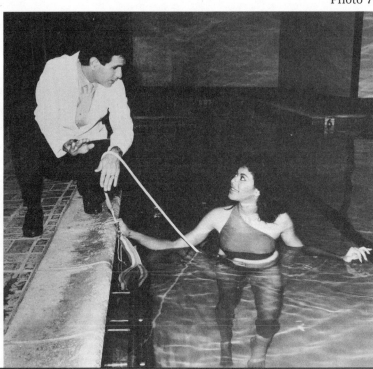

8. WATER RUNNING FOR CONDITIONING WHILE INJURED

Running is **the** universal conditioning activity. Athletes from every sport use it as a primary method of increasing their strength, speed, and stamina—for improving their competitive performances. So it should be no surprise to any injured athlete that water running is becoming the heart of water rehabilitation programs: Following most injuries the athlete can go directly into water and run to maintain and improve overall conditioning. That's because running in water is nontraumatic. There is no pounding on a solid surface.

Mary Decker Slaney, America's foremost middle-distance runner, has had incredible results from water running. Leg injuries and stress breakdowns have plagued her for the past decade. Several weeks prior to the 1984 Olympic Games she suffered from such a painful Achilles' tendon that she limped even when walking in chest-deep water. The task of Mary and of her coach Dick Brown became the quick rehabilitation of Mary's tendon at the same time that she built her overall fitness level toward an Olympic peak. Imagination was called for in 92° water (the standard temperature of a therapy pool).

Dick had Mary run suspended in water as she had been doing in her water training program for the past two years, only now she used a new four-sided suspension system for increased bouyancy, the Aqua Ark. She added 3-pound weight gloves and wore her running flats for a little extra weight. To increase the demand on her cardiovascular system, Mary's available oxygen was restricted by wearing a mask and breathing apparatus that simulates running at an altitude of 7200 feet. Thus outfitted, Mary ran workouts of speed and time lengths that sought duplication of her intense workouts on land. So successful were these "land-equivalent" workouts, .together with one cortisone shot and her daily Acuscope treatments, Mary was able to run a world record 2000 meters after

continued on page 132

only a single land speed workout following her water training.

Mary entered her 1984 Olympic 3000 meter race feeling as strong and fast as she ever had in her life.

In photo 8A coach Dick Brown works with Olympian Bill McChesney who trains suspended in the Aqua Ark. Bill wears the same PO_2 tanks Mary Decker Slaney wore.

Photo 8A

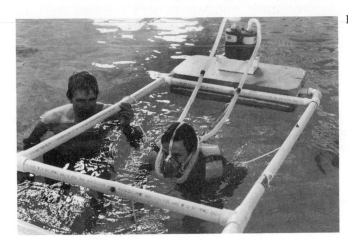

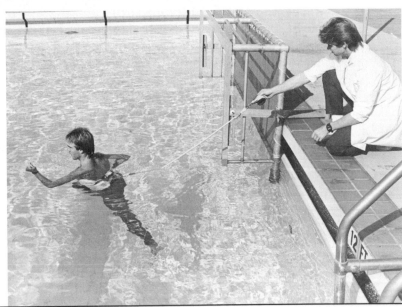

Photo 8B

Strapped in a flotation belt (photo 8B), this runner's feet will never meet the bottom of the pool. He is a high school basketball player with patellar tendinitis ("jumper's knee"). He's working with Dr. Vicky Vodon, who holds him on a tether while she teaches him correct running form in the water. When the athlete is comfortable with driving his arms and legs directly forward and backward (with no lateral deviations), Dr. Vodon can attach her end of the tether to one side of the pool and let him continue alone.

He starts with a 10-minute warm-up of slow, steady running. Next, he watches the wall clock or his waterproof wristwatch to time himself for a series of 15 second sprints. He'll sprint 15, jog and recover 15 until he has done 10 such intervals. His water running ends with 5 minutes of fartlek (see page 108), as he mentally reenacts the normal rhythm of a basketball game.

As his knee improves with exercise over the next weeks, Dr. Vodon removes one of the flotation belts and allows him to run lightly on the bottom of the pool with the minimum support that one belt gives him. The next step in this gradual weight-bearing increase is to let the athlete run without flotation devices, with only the support of chest-deep water and then shallower water. Finally, the basketball player can return to the gym and to his sport. To keep his shooting and reaction skills sharp, the athlete can do Sport-Specific Water Training exercises 3 and 4 during his rehabilitation.

9. WATER PARCOURSE

Dr. Mike Greenberg has combined tethered running and tethered swimming with six other water exercises in an experimental parcourse program for injured athletes—The Seven Seas Gym. Athletes move from station to station around the pool just as they do around a parcourse on land, doing reps, sets, and minutes on a stopwatch at each station, then moving on in a preplanned pattern.

At the first station the athletes warm up by running straight legged, suspended on tethers (photo 9A). Notice that these two athletes are using their arms in a normal running motion but their legs stay straight throughout in order to strengthen their lower back and gluteals, and to warm up their hamstrings for sprinting later. Ankle weights can be added to build the upper quads, psoas, and lower abdominals, but the added weight has to be compensated for: The runner must wear a second flotation belt. After the warm-up, athletes move on to train and have fun with a tethered punching bag, a rowing machine (only the head is above water), an underwater gym (balance beam, rings, and an incline board for inverted sit-ups), a Nordic ski simulator, a free weights station, and then back to tethers for swimming and running distances and sprints.

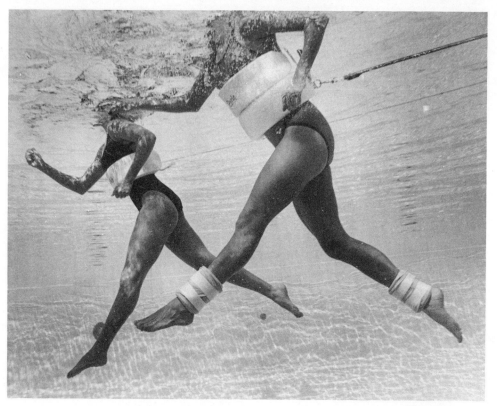

Photo 9A

Seven Seas aftercare includes poolside treatment with Acuscope and Myopulse, which 1984 Olympian Ruth Wysocki receives in photo 9B.

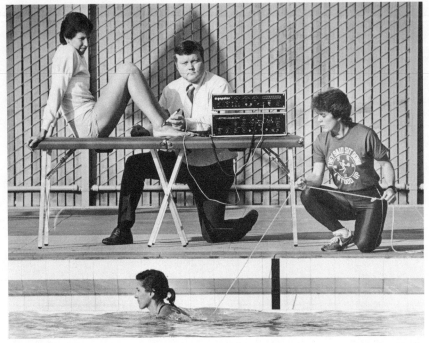

Photo 9B

9
ARTHRITIS WATER THERAPY

August 1981: Sea Cliff, Long Island, New York

For over a week I had been writing a series of radio broadcasts with sportswriter R. R. Knudson (Zan) at her beach house. I noticed that each morning Zan typed with difficulty, but that her hands became increasingly mobile over the course of the day. She told me that arthritis "worked" that way, that her joints were stiff in the mornings, but loosened up later.

While we worked, I looked out a wall-sized window at Long Island Sound. Right there in front of her house Zan had a built-in saltwater healing unit. I took her into the warm water the next morning and we both did water stretches after which we simply walked 10 minutes in waist-deep salt water. Zan shook her hands, stretched them, squeezed them, then massaged them underwater. A skeptic at first, she had to admit that her fingers and other joints moved more easily.

Arthritis causes deterioration of various joint structures, resulting in inflammation, pain, immobilization, and loss of function. It is a degenerative joint condition often caused by excessive or faulty mechanical forces on joints, heredity, faulty calcium metabolism, or more likely a combination of all these factors.

For years the accepted theory was that injured or impaired joints should be rested, but today that theory is considered incorrect, for now it is understood that joints must move to regain their health and integrity. Movement stimulates the synovial lining of all joints to produce synovial fluid, which washes through the entire joint capsule, bringing in fresh nutrients and taking out waste products. This cleansing process reduces swelling and facilitates healing of joint tissue.

All joints are surrounded by muscles and tendons, so for efficient and stable joint function, it is important that these structures be strong. Strong muscles and tendons help joints support the body during weightbearing. But when muscles are allowed to become weak through disuse, they cannot lend support to troubled joints.

Thus for joints to have the greatest chance for health, they must **move,** and the surrounding muscles and tendons must be strong.

Dr. Vicky Vodon, Director of the Chiropractic Health and Sports Care Center in Huntington Beach, California, sees dozens of arthritis patients each week. As the personal doctor and trainer for Olympic gold-medalist Evelyn Ashford and other world-class athletes, Dr. Vodon focuses on helping each athlete or patient achieve maximum performance from his or her body. She expects no less from arthritis patients.

Dr. Vodon's treatment plan for those with arthritis diseases starts with nutritional counseling followed by water therapy in hot and cold whirlpool contrast baths to increase circulation as in photos 1A and 1B. Finally, the patient starts a water exercise program to increase range of motion in all joints and to strengthen all the muscles of the body, particularly those surrounding the arthritis joints. See photos 2A and 2B.

This stretching and strengthening program takes place in water because water's support for the body eliminates the trauma of weight bearing, and water's massaging quality

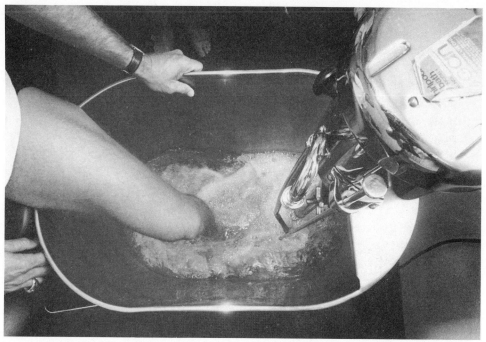

Photo 1A

*Ice cold (1A) and hot (1B) contrast whirlpool baths
reduce inflammation, swelling, and pain in arthritic joints.*

Photo 1B

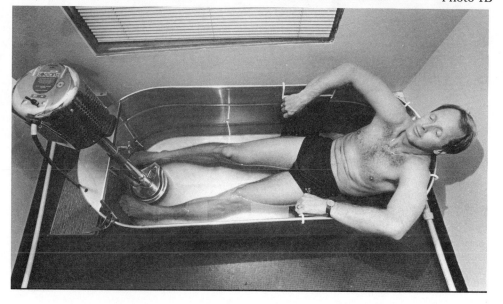

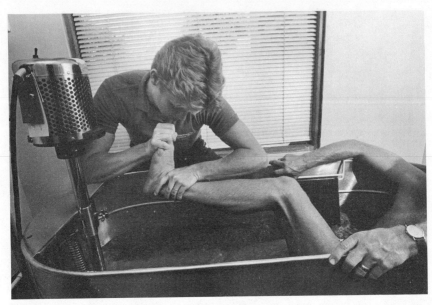

Photo 2A   *Dr. Vodon eases this arthritic ankle (2A), knee and hip (2B) into an increased range of motion.*   Photo 2B

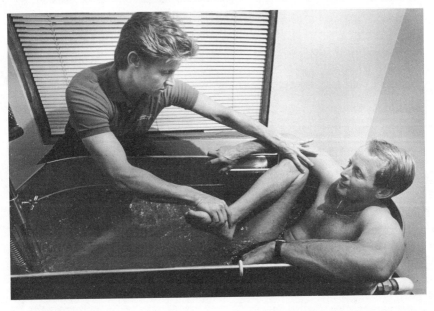

helps the body relax, counteracting the energy-draining effects of chronic pain.

When you do the Arthritis Water Therapy programs in this chapter, observe these general principles:

- Choose a time for your exercise program that will be the best time of day for you—when you are most flexible and energetic. Do as many reps as you can **without strain.**
- Rest whenever you feel fatigued. Tired muscles don't provide adequate support for arthritic joints.
- Move affected joints through a full range of motion at least once a day—in the shower or bathtub if you can't get to a pool.
- Start each exercise routine slowly, with care. Work into each stretch or exercise gradually.
- Strive for an even rhythm in your water therapy routine, for rhythmic exercise is known to produce natural pain-killers in the body and therefore has a tranquilizing effect.
- Always move body parts toward a normal position, especially if joint instability has caused any deformity or deviation in structure or function.
- Learn to distinguish the difference between the usual discomfort of moving arthritic joints and the pain caused by improper alignment or excessive demand on a joint. Continuing an exercise in the presence of sudden or severe pain is likely to cause further joint damage.
- Plan on improving your physical condition. Using Arthritis Water Therapy under your doctor's supervision will cause your symptoms to **decrease,** while your strength, mobility, and vitality will **increase.**

  Work toward the time you'll be regularly using water workouts and swimming, nonweight-bearing activities, as your major fitness tool.

If you experience chronic pain due to arthritis, you are probably not highly motivated to exercise. Movement most likely causes you pain, fatigue, and perhaps even fear and depression. Yet movement is necessary if you wish to stop the degenerating effects of arthritis.

If you've been sedentary because of arthritis, begin your water therapy program in your nightly bath. Add Epsom salts to the hot water to reduce inflammation. Do exercises 2 through 12 from Chapter 10 (pages 148–159) to begin strengthening weak muscles and stretching tight ones.

Once your doctor has approved more strenuous water exercise, find a warm pool and walk around in the water 3 to 5 minutes. Then do the Water Stretch Exercises in Chapter 3 (pages 28–36). Dr. Vodon recommends a minimum water temperature of 86° and a minimum air temperature of 78°.

After doing Water Stretch twice a week for a month, you will probably feel very confident in the water, and may even be eager for a more vigorous routine. If so, do the following exercises:

1. Poolside Flutter Kick (See Exercise 11, page 53.)
2. Scissors (See Exercise 12, page 54.)
3. Knees to Chest Twist (See Exercise 13, page 54.)
4. Paddling—all variations (See Exercise 15, pages 56–58.)
5. Twister (See Exercise 16, page 59.)
6. Lateral Leg Raises (See Exercise 17, page 60.)
7. Hamstring Curls (See Exercise 18, page 61.)
8. Leg Swings (See Exercise 20, page 63.)

After doing these exercises, walk around in the pool at your own pace. Gently rotate, twist, bend, or stretch any part of your body that still aches. If you know how to swim, begin with several lengths of the pool, gradually adding more each workout until you are swimming for 10 minutes.

End your water therapy session with a pain-free float. Nonswimmers can put on a life vest or flotation device. Lean back, and enjoy the wonders of water.

ARTHRITIS WATER THERAPY WORKOUT

1. POOLSIDE FLUTTER KICK

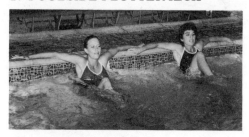

2. SCISSORS

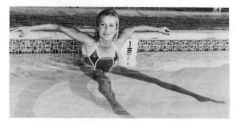

3. KNEES TO CHEST TWIST

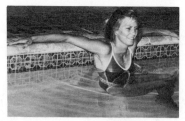

4. PADDLING
Lateral

Pull down, lift behind

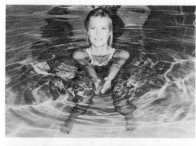
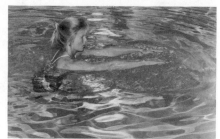

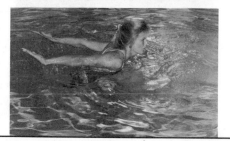

continued on page 144

4. PADDLING *continued*
Downward, upward

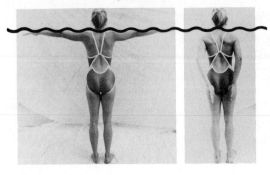

5. TWISTER

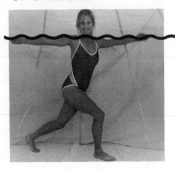

6. LATERAL LEG RAISES

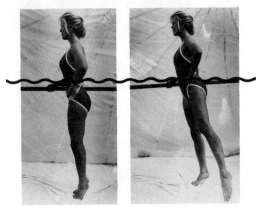

7. HAMSTRING CURLS

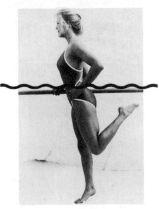

8. LEG SWINGS

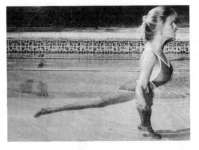

10
PRENATAL WATERPOWER

The fitness activity best suited for pregnancy is exercising in water. Exercise on land raises your body temperature, which activates the body's automatic cooling system. Circulation is then directed to the surface of the skin, away from the fetus, limiting the nourishment that can reach the fetus. Exercising in water keeps the body's temperature down during even the most strenuous workout. Further, the water supports your increasing weight and also extends your range of motion, making all your movements easier: You'll feel weightless and athletic in a pool. As you gain pound after pound during pregnancy and lose sight of your former figure, both your mind and your body will relish the time spent in water. There you will strengthen your muscles, gain all-around flexibility, improve your endurance, and relieve tension. Remember, always consult your doctor before beginning any prenatal fitness program.

In this chapter, you will find instructions for two workouts—one for the tub and one for the pool.

Do these exercises at least 3 times a week throughout your pregnancy.

PRENATAL BATHTUB WORKOUT

Your bathtub is the perfect place for a water workout. It's right in your own home, it's deep enough to submerge your legs, it's long enough for you to stretch them, and it's wide enough to bend your knees to the sides. Your movements will be unrestricted by a bathing suit. Further, you can control the water's temperature (warm, not intensely hot) and also control the time of day or night you enter the water for approximately a 20-minute workout.

Exercises 1 through 12 will give you a moderate warm-up, a good stretch, and key movements for strengthening the abdominals and thighs—all in about 20 minutes. On days when you find it difficult to leave the house, draw a bath, warm up with the cross crawl, and discover a new source for Waterpower.

Evelyn Ashford, pictured in this chapter, is a 1984 Olympic double gold medalist. She is 4 months pregnant in the photos.

Exercise 1 CROSS CRAWL

Stand erect. Lift your pubic bone, which forces you to tuck your tailbone down. Now lift your right arm and left knee (photo 1). Lower them as you lift your left arm and right knee. Using a comfortable pace, do 15 right-left cycles standing in place. Inhale the first time you raise the right hand. Exhale the next time you raise your right hand.

This exercise warms most of your major muscle groups.

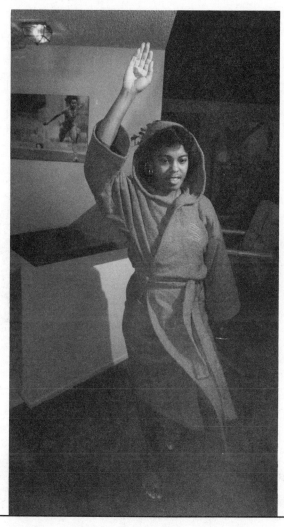

Photo 1

Exercise 2 FEET UNDER FAUCET

When the bathtub is about half full, sit down and place your feet under the water that is running to fill the tub (photo 2). Rotate your ankles clockwise, then counterclockwise. Your added weight during pregnancy puts pressure on your feet and cuts down circulation, which causes swelling. The massaging effect of the warm water speed circulation and reduces swelling.

Photo 2

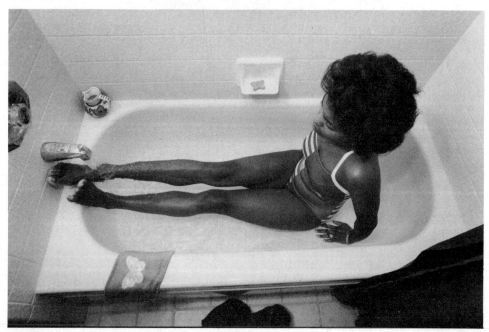

Exercise 3 RELAX AND BREATHE

Lean back in a comfortable position. Begin breathing in a slow and deliberate way, concentrating on each breath. Breathe deeply and allow your abdomen to rise as you inhale (photo 3). Push that breath out using your stomach muscles. Keep pushing with the stomach muscles until you've squeezed out as much air as you can. Now inhale to a count of 4, hold your breath for 2 counts, and once again push your breath out by contracting your stomach muscles. The ability to control your breathing in a calm, deliberate way will be necessary during childbirth.

Continue 3 to 5 minutes.

Photo 3

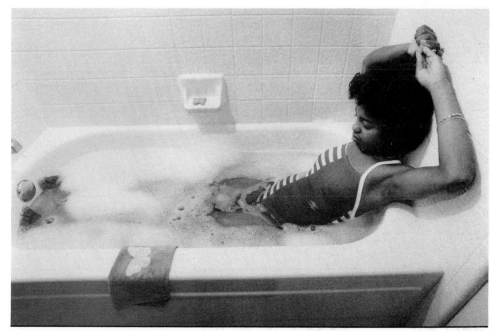

Exercise 4 FORWARD BEND

With your knees slightly bent, reach forward and comfortably place both hands on your feet, ankles, or shins. Drop your chin and let your head hang comfortably forward (photo 4). Breathe deeply 10 times, remembering to use your abdominals with each exhalation. As you do this, the forceful abdominal contractions strengthen your stomach, and the forward bend stretches your lower back. Low-back flexibility should be emphasized during pregnancy so that the back doesn't become overly strong in relation to the abdominals, causing low-back pain.

Now increase the water in the tub so that the warmth comes up at least to your waist.

Photo 4

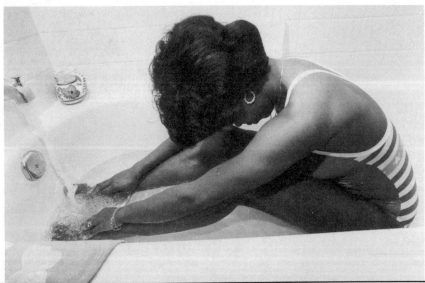

Exercise 5 BENT KNEE SIDE TWIST

Bend your left knee, bringing your left foot to your right inner thigh. Place your right hand on your left knee for leverage. Twist to your left, reaching your left arm over your head toward your right foot (photo 5).

Repeat with your right foot on your left inner thigh.

Your hips are submerged in warm water, which aids the stretch. Hip and groin flexibility will be crucial during delivery of your baby, so become aware of any muscle tightness that may be in your hips. If you feel such tightness, inhale deeply, visualizing the breath going to the problem area. Try to unclench the muscle as you exhale.

Photo 5

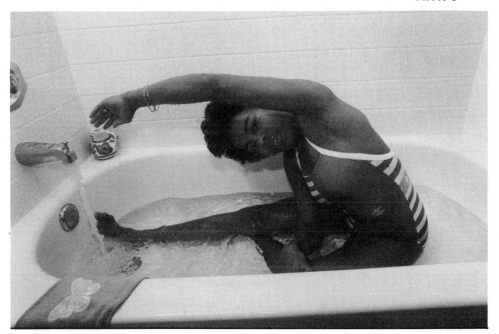

Exercise 6 SPINAL TWIST

Legs and feet point straight ahead throughout this exercise. Lift your chest, then twist to the left. Hold on to the edge of the bathtub with both hands (photo 6). With each exhalation, lift and twist even further. Contract your abdominals on each exhalation, holding your position and relaxing your back muscles. Continue to lift, twist, and hold for five deep breaths, then repeat the entire process twisting to the right. If you can't hold on to the tub, put your hands on the tile for leverage.

Now slide down onto your back with water covering your body for a moment. Relax and breathe, using the ratio inhale 4, hold 2, exhale 8 counts.

Photo 6

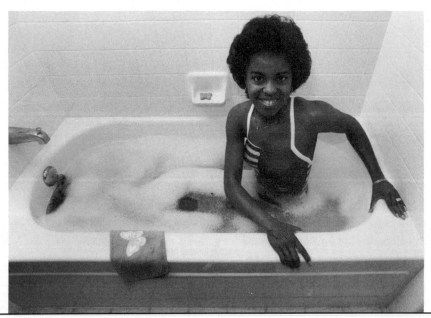

Exercise 7 LEG OPENERS

Both legs remain straight ahead but are now on the surface of the water. Brace yourself as in photo 7A. Your back is rounded, taking pressure off your lower back. Open (photo 7B) and close your legs 25 times. Choose your own level of work: If you move slowly, there will be little water resistance; if you move quickly and forcefully, you will dramatically increase your workload.

Adductors (inner thigh muscles) stabilize your pelvis and are necessary in developing abdominal strength. Both adductors and abdominals are strengthened in this exercise without undue strain because the water helps you hold your legs up as you move them laterally.

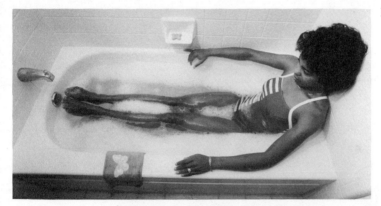

Photo 7A

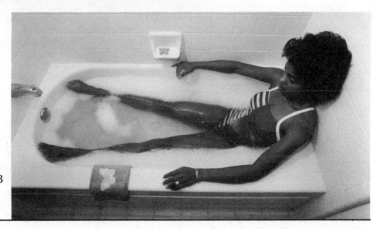

Photo 7B

Exercise 8 SINGLE LEG EXTENSIONS

Your lower back is rounded as you clasp both hands around your right knee and pull it toward your chest. Now extend your left leg just above the surface of the water (photo 8). Hold this position while you inhale 4 counts, hold your breath 2 counts, and exhale 8 counts, contracting your stomach muscles on each exhalation. If you begin to feel strain in your lower back, stop and reposition yourself, making sure your lower back is rounded. Start again. Repeat with the left knee to your chest and the right leg extended.

As you gain strength, do 3 to 5 breathing cycles on one leg before switching to the other leg.

Photo 8

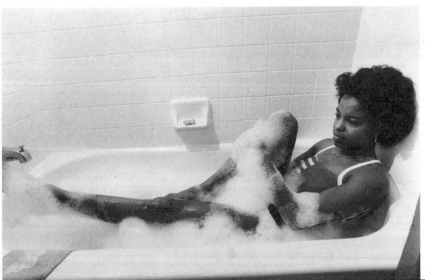

Exercise 9 DOUBLE LEG EXTENSIONS

Keep your lower back rounded and use both arms to brace yourself in the tub. Inhale and pull both knees toward your chest (photo 9A). With an exhale, contract your stomach muscles fully, straighten both legs, and point your toes toward the ceiling (photo 9B). Inhale-bend, then exhale-straighten 15 times.

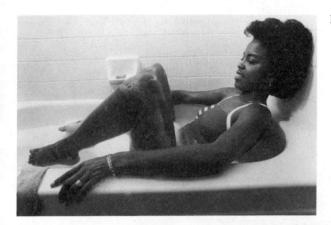

Photo 9A

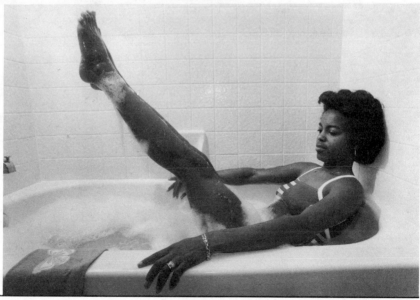

Photo 9B

continued on page 156

Now hold your legs up in the straight position shown in photo 9B. Flex your feet toward your head (photo 9C). Point and flex 15 times. Be sure your knees are straight for maximum stretch of calf and thigh. The stretch of the hamstring is aided by the warm water surrounding it.

In your last trimester of pregnancy, you will probably have to open your legs in all positions of this exercise—bent, straight, pointed, flexed (photo 9D).

Slide down and relax.

Photo 9C

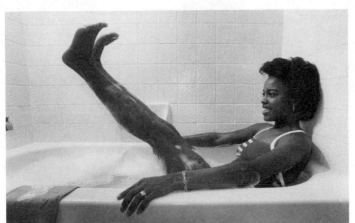

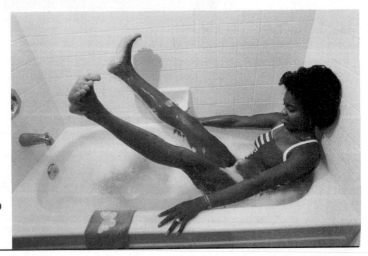

Photo 9D

Exercise 10 GROIN STRETCH

Try the advanced stretch in photo 10A only if you already have reasonably good groin and inner thigh flexibility. Otherwise, go directly to the exercise shown in photo 10B.

Put your hands on the edge of the tub for support and lower yourself as far as you are comfortable (photo 10A). Breathe deeply 5 times, using your abdominal muscles. With each exhalation you will probably feel yourself easing lower into the water.

Now assume the position in photo 10B. Bring the soles of your feet together with your knees out to each side. Inhale 4 counts, hold 2 counts, and exhale 8 counts. Gradually increase the force of your abdominal contractions as each exhalation progresses. Do these breathing exercises in the groin stretch position (photo 10B) 3 to 5 minutes.

Inner thigh, groin, and hip flexibility is of primary importance in delivery.

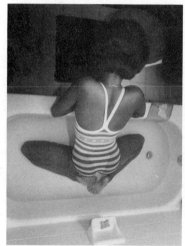

Photo 10A

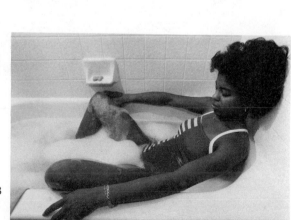

Photo 10B

Exercise 11 CALF AND ACHILLES' STRETCH

Stand up in the tub and brace yourself with both hands against a wall. Bend your right knee and straighten your left leg behind you (photo 11), thus stretching your left calf and Achilles' tendon.

Ankles tend to swell during pregnancy. Stretching them as you do with this exercise helps stimulate circulation, keeping you mobile.

Exercise 12 SHOULDER STRETCH WITH TOWEL

Stand up straight and hold a small towel in your right hand. Lift your right elbow and place your right hand behind your neck. Bend your left arm behind your back and grasp the towel. Now pull down gently with your left hand in order to stretch the right shoulder (photo 12). Switch hands. Repeat several times as the water drains from the tub.

Your posture is important during this exercise. Tuck your tailbone down to keep yourself from becoming swaybacked.

Photo 11

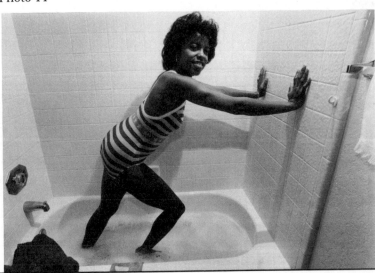

Breathing Correctly

As you dry yourself after this workout, think over the rhythmic method of breathing recommended in most of these exercises. Emphasis has been on slow, deliberate breaths that are controlled and synchronized with the movements being done. Emphasis has also been placed on the use of abdominal force with each slow exhalation. Each time you do your workout, establish this same rhythm of breathing that goes smoothly with each exercise. Continue to use forceful abdominal contractions while exhaling. This thoughtful breathing will keep you calm, more efficient in your movements, and better prepared for childbirth.

Photo 12

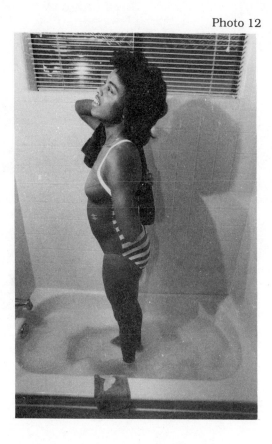

PRENATAL BATHTUB WORKOUT

1. CROSS CRAWL   15 reps

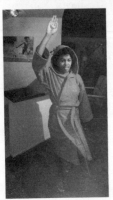

2. FEET UNDER FAUCET
2 minutes

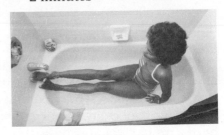

3. RELAX AND BREATHE
3–5 minutes

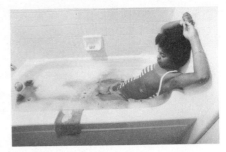

4. FORWARD BEND
2 reps of 5 breaths

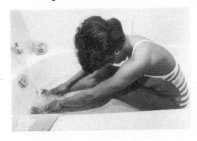

5. BENT KNEE SIDE TWIST
5 breaths each side

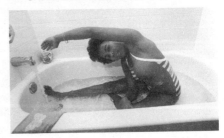

6. SPINAL TWIST
5 breaths each side

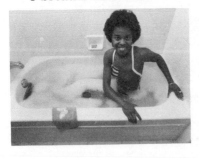

7. *LEG OPENERS* 25 reps

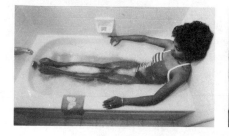 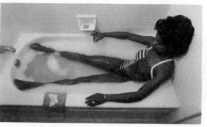

8. *SINGLE LEG EXTENSIONS*
3–5 breaths each side

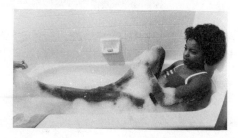

9. *DOUBLE LEG EXTENSIONS* 15 reps

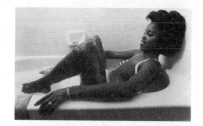 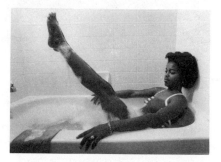

Feet point and flex—15 reps

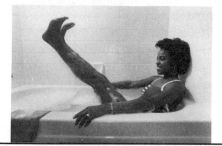 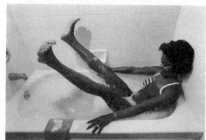

continued on page 162

PRENATAL BATHTUB WORKOUT continued

10. *GROIN STRETCH* 3–5 minutes

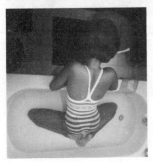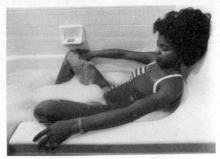

11. *CALF AND ACHILLES' STRETCH*
30 sec each side

12. *SHOULDER STRETCH WITH TOWEL*
30 sec each side

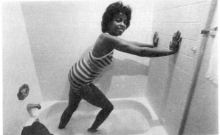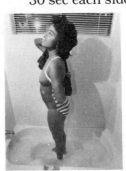

PRENATAL POOL WORKOUT

The following workout will give you light cardiovascular exercise and help you substantially increase your flexibility and the strength of the muscle groups you need most during labor—your abdominals and inner thigh muscles. The complete workout takes about 20 minutes.

Before you enter the pool, do Shower Cool-downs (see pages 24–25). **Do not use Shower Warm-ups 1 and 2. Warm-up 1 is the exact opposite of the posture you are striving for during pregnancy. Warm-up 2 would be uncomfortable in the later months of pregnancy.**

Begin your workout by walking across the pool in chest-deep water, constantly correcting your posture. Lift your head. Lift your shoulders. Lift your pubic bone. Try to keep your tailbone tucked under throughout these exercises (and throughout the day). Standing and walking swayback is the most common cause of lower back pain during pregnancy.

After 5 minutes of walking, try an easy jog. The water will support the extra weight of your breasts and growing baby. Jog until you are comfortable in the pool's temperature (about 2 minutes) and then do these Water Stretch exercises:

1. Tuck and Stretch (See Exercise 1, page 28.)
2. Shoulder Stretch (See Exercise 2, page 29.)
3. Triangle (See Exercise 3, page 30.)
4. Quad Stretch (hold side of pool for support) (See Exercise 6, page 33.)
5. Hamstring Stretch (modify by placing leg 45 degrees to outside) (See Exercise 8, page 35.)

Continue immediately with these exercises from the Basic Water Workout:

6. Poolside Flutter Kick—all variations (See Exercise 11, page 53.)
7. Scissors (See Exercise 12, page 54.)
8. Paddling—all variations (See Exercise 15, pages 56–58.)
9. Twister (See Exercise 16, page 59.)
10. Lateral Leg Raises (See Exercise 17, page 60.)
11. Hamstring Curls (See Exercise 18, page 61.)
12. Quad Extensions (See Exercise 19, page 62.)

After one session, think over your pool experience. Your conclusions just might make your future workouts more pleasurable and purposeful.

First of all, think about the temperature of the water. Did you feel warm enough after 5 minutes or so of exercise and did you stay warm until your final exercise? If not, try going through the exercises faster on your second workout—and a little faster and a little faster, as needed for warmth. Ask the pool director if other users of the pool mention the cold water or if you are alone in doing so. Perhaps after several days of increasing your speed, yet still feeling chilly, you may wish to seek a warmer pool.

Think about your bathing suit. Was it supportive yet loose enough for comfort through your full range of motion? If not, borrow or buy one that is. Also think about your body moving in the pool. Did your exercise form match the photographs in Water Stretch and Waterpower? You might wish to take along a training partner for your next workout so that he or she can read the exercises aloud and check your posture and form against the photos.

Finally, think about your breathing. Did you choke on swallowed water because you took a breath at the wrong moment in the exercise? Were you winded at any point in the sequence of exercises? Did you catch yourself hyperventilating (taking rapid, shallow breaths) when you should have maintained slower, more rhythmic, more efficient breathing? If your answers are yes to these questions, you may need to work on breathing correctly (see page 159). Also make sure your mouth and nose are well out of the water when you inhale.

PRENATAL POOL WORKOUT

SHOWER COOL-DOWN

CLASP-HANDS-BEHIND-BACK STRETCH
5 breaths

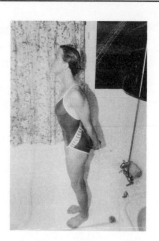

RAG DOLL 5 breaths
Bend Knees, Bend Forward—5 breaths
Walk 5 minutes
Jog 2 minutes

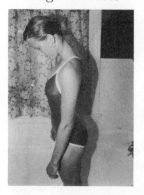 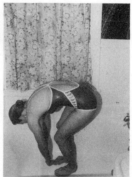

1. TUCK AND STRETCH 1 minute

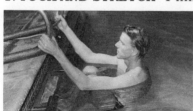

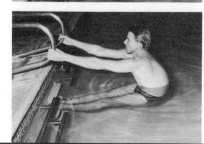

2. SHOULDER STRETCH
1 minute

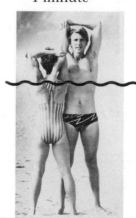

continued on page 166

PRENATAL POOL WORKOUT continued

3. TRIANGLE 1 minute

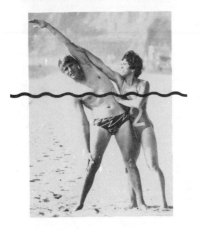

4. QUAD STRETCH 1 minute

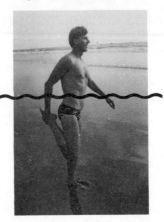

5. HAMSTRING STRETCH 1 minute

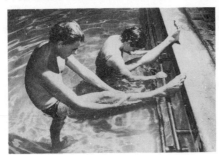

Move leg 45° to right from position pictured to avoid pressure on stomach.

6. POOLSIDE FLUTTER KICK

Back with bicycle, then straight legs—25 reps each
Front with bent, then straight legs—25 reps each

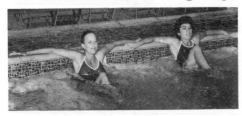

7. SCISSORS 15 reps

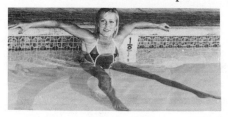

8. PADDLING

Lateral—15 reps

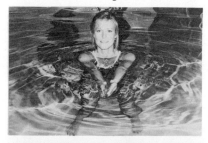

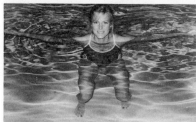

Pull down, lift behind—15 reps

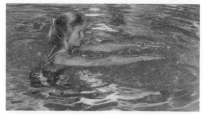

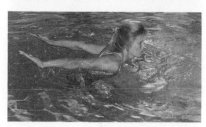

Downward, upward—15 reps

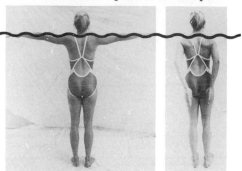

continued on page 168

PRENATAL POOL WORKOUT continued

9. TWISTER 10 reps

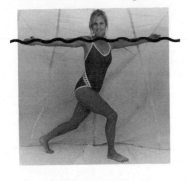

10. LATERAL LEG RAISES 15 reps

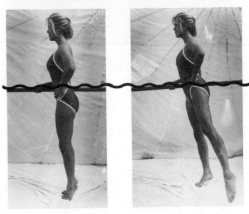

11. HAMSTRING CURLS
15 reps each side

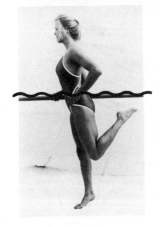

12. QUAD EXTENSIONS 15 reps each side

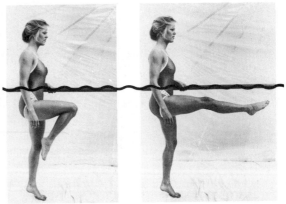

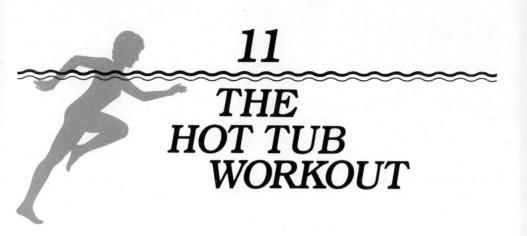

11
THE
HOT TUB
WORKOUT

Hot water power! In a spa, the hot-water jets will help relax muscles that have tightened with fatigue or strain. Comfortably submerged, your veins and arteries dilate, allowing heat to escape. Thus the body maintains temperature equilibrium: Give it heat and it reacts by cooling down.

Give your body also this short series of rejuvenating movements in the hot tub. These movements will:

- Relieve mental stress by changing your focus from work to warm water
- Stretch your major muscle groups
- Supply you with perhaps your only exercise session of the day

Slowly lower yourself into the hot water. Breathe deeply, even sigh out loud as your body releases tension. There will be ledges of various depth in the hot tub. Choose the water level that makes you most comfortable for each of these exercises.

SOLO PROGRAM—Approximately 10 minutes

Exercise 1 LIFT CHIN, DROP CHIN
Trapezius, sternocleidomastoids

Stand, kneel, or sit squarely in the hot tub. Lift your chin toward the ceiling (photo 1). Relax your shoulders and breathe deeply and slowly five times. Now bring your chin to your chest, relax your shoulders, and breathe deeply and slowly five times. Always remember to make your exhalation slower and longer than your inhalation for maximum calming. Repeat both positions one more time.

Exercise 2 CLASP-HANDS-BEHIND-BACK STRETCH
Traps, rhomboids

Stand or sit on the edge of the spa's submerged ledge in water up to your shoulders. Interlace your fingers behind your back and straighten your arms. Pull your shoulders back, squeezing your shoulder blades together (photo 2). Hold this position as you breathe deeply five times. Relax, then repeat, gently twisting from side to side.

Photo 1

Photo 2

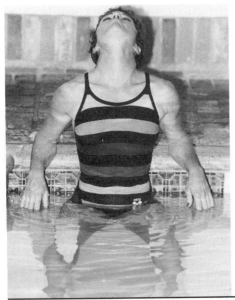
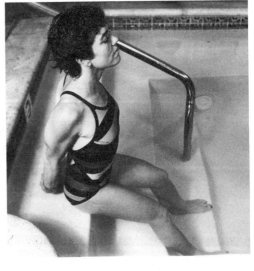

Exercise 3 ARM CURLS TO SIDE

Biceps, triceps, pectorals, latissimus dorsi

While sitting on a ledge or kneeling in the middle of the hot tub, place your arms in the position in photo 3A. Curl your arms through the position shown in photo 3B until your hands touch your chest. Keep your upper arms stationary; only the lower arms move. Elbows remain straight out to the sides. Keep fingers together for maximum water resistance. Repeat 25 times.

Photo 3A

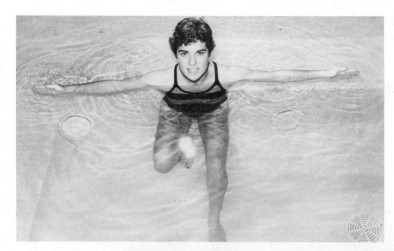

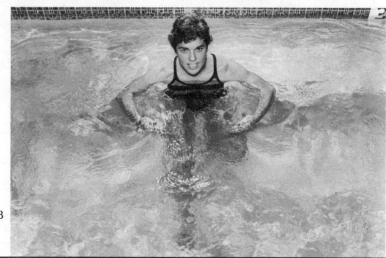

Photo 3B

Before continuing this short course, find the most powerful jet in the hot tub. Place your feet directly in front of the jet spray and enjoy the tingling massage. Repeat with your hands, elbows, knees, calves, and other tense or aching body parts. (Swimmers can go under the water and place the back or top of their heads in front of the jet to relieve headaches—or simply for pleasure.)

Exercise 4 FLUTTER KICK
Gluteals, hamstrings, quadriceps, abdominals

Hold on to the ladder, ledge, or side of the hot tub as in photo 4. Now flutter kick. Count 50 kicks, then turn over onto your back and repeat.

Photo 4

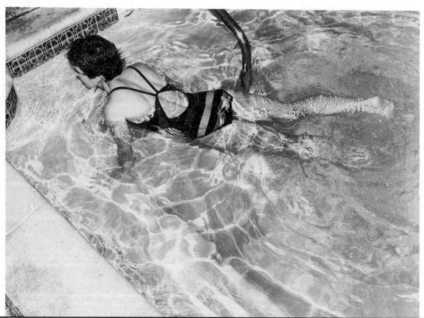

Exercise 5 FLOATING PUSH-UPS

Gluts, hamstrings, triceps, quadratus lumborum

Place your body in a prone position similar to photo 5A, with your lower body relaxed below water level. Now straighten your arms, tighten your buttocks muscles, and attempt to lift both legs behind you above the surface of the water (photo 5B). Your heels will break the water first. Relax. Repeat 10 times.

Before continuing, soak for a few minutes.

Photo 5A

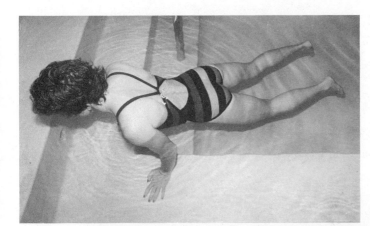

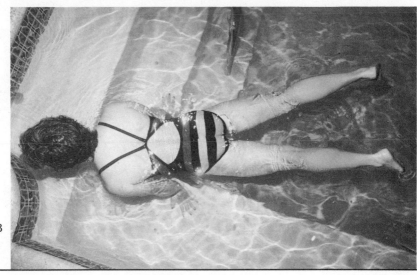

Photo 5B

Exercise 6 SCISSORS

Abductors, adductors

Sit on the edge of the hot tub's submerged ledge. Extend both legs in front of you. Open your legs wide (photo 6A), then cross and recross them, alternating top leg (photo 6B). Repeat 15 times.

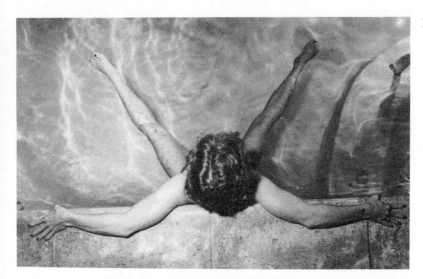

Photo 6A

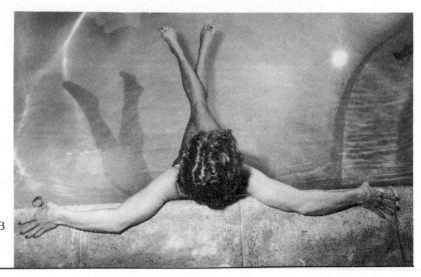

Photo 6B

If you have a hot tub companion, add these exercises:

PARTNER PROGRAM—Approximately 15 minutes

Exercise 7 FORWARD BEND WITH PARTNER
Hamstrings, quadratus lumborum

STRETCHER: Extend both legs straight in front of you while sitting on the submerged ledge. Reach forward toward your feet with both hands. Breathe deeply and relax.

PUSHER: Assume a back-to-back position with your partner. Lean back slowly, pushing your partner forward with a gradual steady pressure. (See photo 7.) Keep your knees bent for balance. Increase or decrease your push according to your partner's instructions. Ease off slowly. Exchange positions.

Photo 7

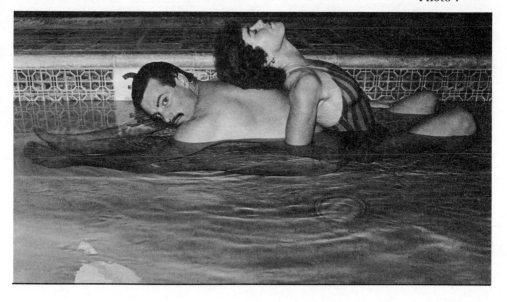

Exercise 8 V-SIT FORWARD BEND WITH PARTNER
Hamstrings, quadratus lumborum, adductors

Find a corner of the hot tub where you and your partner can assume the position in photo 8.

STRETCHER: Open your legs to 90 degrees, knees pointing up toward the ceiling. Reach forward with both hands and grasp your partner's wrists. Breathe deeply as you allow your lower back and inner thigh muscles to relax. If you experience any knee pain, bring your legs closer together.

PULLER: Clasp wrists with your partner, then brace your feet against the ledge and your partner's legs as pictured. Lean back slowly. Gradually increase your effort as you pull on your partner's arms, working only until your partner experiences a slight discomfort. Hold the position there and explore the stretch together by joining breathing patterns—inhale and exhale. You will notice the body "let go" and relax during exhalations. After the stretch, push your partner's knees gently together and toward his chest.

Exchange positions.

Photo 8

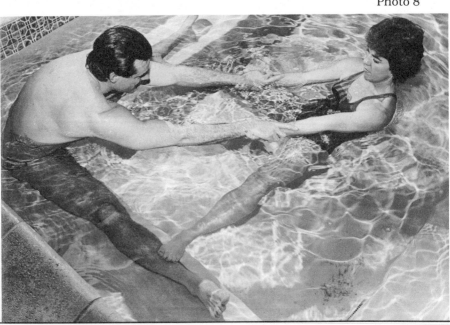

Exercise 9 DOUBLE SHOULDER STRETCH WITH PARTNER

Lats, infraspinatus, teres major and minor

Before beginning this exercise, submerge your body to your chin in hot water. This will help increase the range of motion in your shoulder joints.

STRETCHER: Raise both arms overhead. Allow the weight of your body to pull you downward as your partner pulls up on your hands as in photo 9.

PULLER: Firmly grasp your partner's wrists. Stand in a forward stride, knees bent and tailbone tucked down for stability. Pull upward until your partner feels a slight discomfort. Hold the position until he has taken at least five deep breaths and relaxed comfortably into the position.

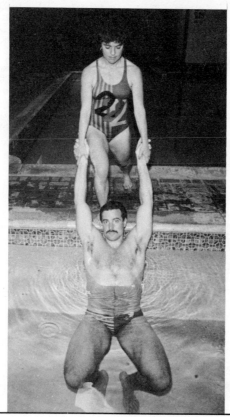

Photo 9

There are several further ways to relax before you leave the hot tub:

- Give yourself or your partner a foot massage (photo 10).
- Lean back against each other (photo 11) and breathe in unison for 3 to 5 minutes.
- Take a deep breath, close your eyes, and begin exhaling through the nose. Lower yourself completely under the water. Continue exhaling, blowing bubbles (photo 12) slowly and gently as long as you comfortably can. Repeat 5 to 10 times as desired for calming and pleasure.

Photo 10

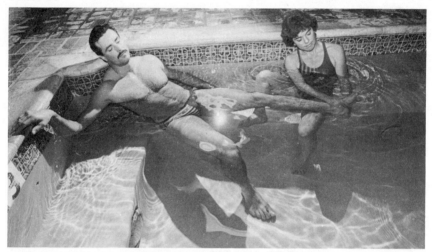

Photo 11

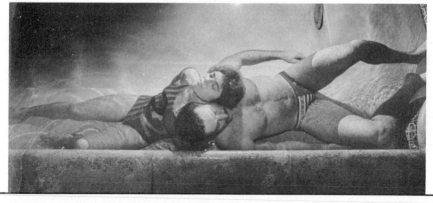

Photo 12

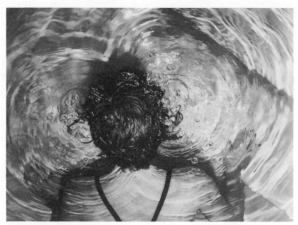

Now take a cool shower and see how invigorated you feel. Your hot tub program can begin your day, interrupt and freshen the routine of your day, or end your day with a relaxed sigh.

HOT TUB WORKOUT

1. LIFT CHIN, DROP CHIN
2 reps, 5 breaths each

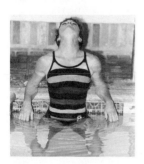

2. CLASP-HANDS-BEHIND-BACK-STRETCH
2 reps, 5 breaths each

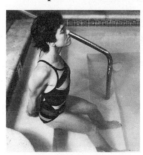

continued on page 180

HOT TUB WORKOUT continued

3. *ARM CURLS TO SIDE* 25 reps—Water jet massage

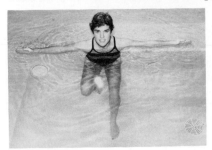 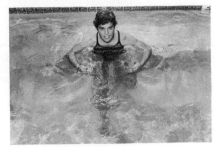

4. *FLUTTER KICK* 50 each, front and back

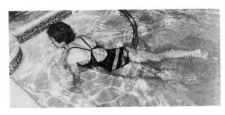

5. *FLOATING PUSH-UPS* 10 reps

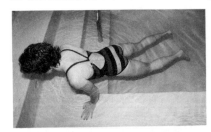 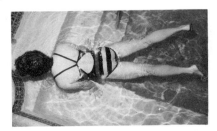

6. *SCISSORS* 15 reps

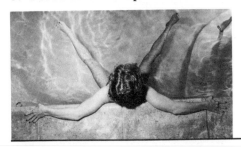 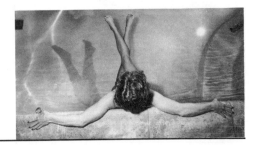

7. *FORWARD BEND WITH PARTNER* 10 breaths

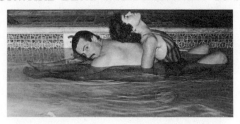

8. *V-SIT FORWARD BEND WITH PARTNER* 10 breaths

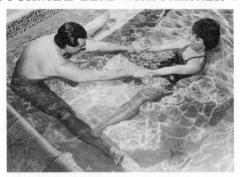

9. *DOUBLE SHOULDER STRETCH WITH PARTNER*
10 breaths

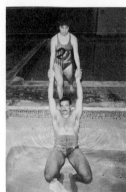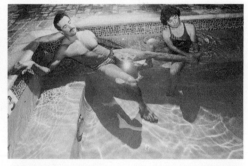

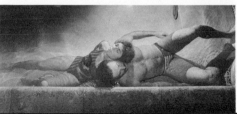

continued on page 182

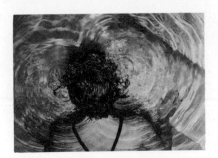

Blow bubbles.

POSTSCRIPT: THE JOY OF WATERPOWER

June 1985: Rome, Italy

My 800 meter race in the World Veterans Track and Field Championships was scheduled for early Saturday evening. When my left Achilles' tendon told me quite loudly that I couldn't race, I figured I had two options: I could stay at the track meet in Rome and mope or I could take to the open water for adventure and strenuous exercise.

Sunday morning I drove south toward Naples and caught the first boat from Pozzouli to the island of Ischia. The water there was clean and clear—20 foot visibility. I swam parallel to the shore past brightly colored hotels and their matching rows of beach chairs and umbrellas. There I got the idea of beach-hopping, swimming in as many bodies of water as I could during my week in Europe. I headed back to the mainland and drove further south past Sorrento; I found Big Sur, Italian style: the gorgeous Amalfi coast. I couldn't resist stopping for an invigorating swim at each lovely cove. Next I traversed Italy from its Mediterranean shore to its Adriatic coastline. From Bari, I took an overnight boat ride to Corfu, Greece. There, in the 50 to 80 foot water visibility of the Ionian Sea, I enjoyed three or four swims a day, hopping all over the island to try out the warmer, cooler, saltier, or clearer waters of each bay.

By the time I returned to Rome, my athletic disappointment had long been forgotten, replaced by the joy of water.

It's taken me many years to develop a fitness life-style that serves me well year in, year out—that also sees me through the heartbreak of injury suffered in the heat of competition or serious training.

The key has been adding water to my varied workouts.

The water has rescued me so many times that I now take it for granted. But if you haven't yet incorporated into your life the joy, the satisfaction, the downright FUN of working out in water, begin now. Once you feel comfortable taking your training into a pool, hot tub, or ocean, the water will become your best training partner. And for the rest of your life you'll be glad, as I am, that water is such a forgiving and dependable friend.

INDEX

Acuscope, 128, 131, 136
Aerobics, water, 6, 69–82
  aerobic water running,
    74
  backstroke on tethers,
    74–75
  cardiovascular fitness
    and, 69–70
  guidelines for, 71
  pool warm-up, 72
  suspended aerobic water
    running, 73
  water circuit training,
    see Water circuit
    training
  working heart rate target
    zones, 72
  workout program, 81
Aerobic sports skills
  exercise, 80
Aerobic water running, 74

Ankle rehabilitation, 7
Aqua Ark, 131, 132
Arm curls to side, 171–72
Arthritis water therapy, 7,
    137–44
  description of arthritis,
    137–38
  movement and, 138, 142
  principles of, 141
  Vondon's treatment for,
    138–41, 142
  workout program, 142–
    44
Ashford, Evelyn, xiv, 138,
    146

Backstroke on tethers, 74–
    75
Baseball exercises, 94–96
  practice baseball swing,
    94

water medicine ball, 95–96

Basic water workout, 5–6, 41–68
  bouncing, 42–43
  dips, 55
  frog jumps, 49
  hamstring curls, 61
  hitch kicks, 46
  intervals, 51
  jump and sprint, 50
  jumping, no arms, 44
  knees to chest twist, 54
  lateral leg raises, 60
  leg swings, 63
  lunges, 45
  paddling, 56–58
  poolside flutter kick, 53
  quad extensions, 62
  rocking horse, 46–47
  scissors, 54
  straddle jumps, 48
  tips for, 41–42
  twister, 59
  water tripping, 52
  workout program, 64–68

Basketball exercises, 96–97
  block shot with drag suit, 97
  jump shot with drag suit, 96

Bathing suits, selecting, 13

Bent knee side twist, 151

Block shot with drag suit, 97

Bouncing, 42–43

Brown, Dick, 131, 132

Calf and Achilles stretch, 158

Calf rehabilitation, 129

Cardiovascular fitness, 69–70
  working heart rate target zones, 72, 75–76

Casey, Bernie, xiv, 15, 90

Catch, 102

Chamberlain, Wilt, xiv, 88, 119–23

Chest rehabilitation, 125

Clasp-hands-behind-back stretch:
  in a hot tub, 170
  in the shower, 24

Concentration, 88–89

Crescent moon, 32

Cross-country skiing exercise, 99

Cross crawl, 147

Curious onlookers, 89

Cycling exercise, 98–99

Dips, 55

Discus exercises, 100–101
  key position practice, 100
  rotation practice, 101

Double leg extensions, 155–56

Elbow rehabilitation, 119–23

Equipment, extra, 13, 16–17

Exercise class, 87

Feet under faucet, 148
Fins, 13
Floating push-ups, 173
Flutter kick, 172
Football/rugby exercises,
    102–103
  catch, 102
  run, no fumble, 103
Forward bend:
  in a hot tub, 175–76
  prenatal, 150
  V-sit, 176
Frog jumps, 49
  moving, 77
  one-legged, 79

Goals:
  keeping, 9–10
  setting, 83–84
Goggles, 13–14
Golf exercises, 104
  partner arm press, 104
  practice swing, 104
Greenberg, Dr. Mike, xv,
    87, 124, 128, 129, 134
Greenberg Float Coat, 14
  backstroke on tethers,
    using, 74–75
Groin stretch, 34
  prenatal, 157

Hamstring curls, 61
Hamstring stretch, 35–36
  in the shower, 23
Harmon, Marlene, xiv, 71,
    85
Having fun, 91
Hitch kicks, 46

Hot tub workout (solo), 8,
    169–74
  arm curls to side, 171–
    72
  clasp-hands-behind-back
    stretch, 170
  floating push-ups, 173
  flutter kick, 172
  lift chin, drop chin, 170
  relaxation tips, 178–79
  scissors, 174
  workout program, 179–
    80
Hot tub workout (with a
    partner), 8, 169, 175–
    77
  double shoulder stretch,
    177
  forward bend, 175
  V-sit forward bend, 176
  workout program, 181–
    82
Huey, Lynda, 15, 117–19,
    183–84

Juantoreno, Alberto, xiv,
    115
Jump and sprint, 50
Jumping, no arms, 44
Jump on command, 110
Jump shot with drag suit,
    96

Key position practice, 100
Kickboard, 14
  water circuit training
    with, 76–77
Knee pull stretch, 31

Knees to chest twist, 54
Knudson, R. R. (Zan), 137

Ladder arm press, 78
Lateral leg raises, 60
Leg openers, 153
Leg swings, 63
Lift chin, drop chin, 170
Lower back rehabilitation,
   126–27
Lunges, 45

McChesney, Bill, 132
Martial arts exercise, 105
Medicine ball, water, 95
Moving frog jumps, 77
Muscles, 11–12
   chart of, 16–17
Myopause, 128, 136

Paddling, 56–58
Partner arm press, 104
Partner leg press, 98–99
Perry Flotation Belt and
   Perry-Band, 14
Pools:
   choosing, 12–13
   ignoring curious
     onlookers, 89
   establishing your
     workout space, 89
Poolside flutter kick, 53
Practice kick, 110
Practice swing:
   golf club, 104
   racket sports, 106
Prenatal bathtub workout,
   7–8, 145–64

bent knee side twist, 151
calf and Achilles' stretch,
   158
cross crawl, 147
double leg extensions,
   155–56
feet under faucet, 148
forward bend, 150
groin stretch, 157
leg openers, 153
relax and breathe, 149
shoulder stretch with
   towel, 158–59
single leg extensions,
   154
spinal twist, 152
workout program, 160–
   62
Prenatal pool workout,
   162–68
Programs, choosing, 4–8

Quad extensions, 62
Quad stretch, 33

Racket sports exercises,
   106–107
   practice swing, 106
   tidal wave, 107
Rag doll, 25
Rehabilitation, water, 6–7,
   115–36
   ankle, 130
   calf, 129
   chest, 125
   elbow, 119–23
   lower back, 126–27
   principles of, 116–17

shoulder, 124
thigh, 128
water parcourse, 134
water running for
    conditioning, 131–33
water's healing powers,
    117–19
Relax and breathe, 149
Rocking horse, 46–47
Rose, Murray, xiv, 3
Rotation practice, 101
Run, no fumble, 103
Running exercise, 108
Running in water for
    conditioning while
    injured, 131–33

Safety tips, 18–19
Scissors, 54
    in a hot tub, 174
Shoulder rehabilitation,
    124
Shoulder stretch, 29
    prenatal, with towel, 158–
    59
Shower exercises, 21–26
    clasp-hands-behind-back
        stretch, 24
    hamstring stretch, 23
    rag doll, 25
    shower pose, 22
    workout program, 26
Shower pose, 22
Side benefits, 90–91
Single leg extensions, 154
Slaney, Mary Decker, 131–
    32
Smith, Tommie, 118

Soccer exercises, 110
    jump on command, 110
    practice kick, 110
Spinal twist, 152
Sport-specific water
    training, 6, 93–114
    baseball, 94–96
    basketball, 96–97
    cross-country skiing, 99
    customizing your
        program, 113
    cycling, 98–99
    discus, 100–101
    equipment for, 14
    football/rugby, 102–103
    golf, 104
    list of, 113–14
    martial arts, 105
    racket sports, 106–107
    running, 108
    soccer, 110
    volleyball, 112
Sprinting on tether, 108
Starke, George, 118
Straddle jumps, 48
Stretch, water, 5, 27–40
    crescent moon, 32
    groin stretch, 34
    hamstring stretch, 35–
    36
    improving your workout,
    37
    knee pull stretch, 31
    quad stretch, 33
    shoulder stretch, 29
    triangle, 30
    tuck and stretch, 28
    workout program, 37–
    40

Stride practice, 99
Suspended aerobic water running, 73

Thigh rehabilitation, 128
Tidal wave, 107
Tips for improved waterpower, 83–91
  concentrate, 88–89
  establish a workout schedule, 84–86
  establish your workout space in the pool, 89
  have fun, 91
  ignore curious onlookers, 89
  keep your goals firmly in mind, 83–84
  notice side benefits, 90–91
  training partner or exercise class, 86–87
Training partner, 86–87
Tree pose, 105
Triangle, 30
Tuck and stretch, 28
Twister, 59

Van Wolvelaere, Patty, 1
Volleyball exercise, 112
Vondon, Dr. Vicky, xv, 17, 125, 133, 138–41, 142

Water circuit training, 75–82
  aerobic sports skills, 80
  kickboard, 76–77
  ladder arm press, 78
  moving frog jumps, 77
  one-legged frog jumps, 79
  working heart rate and, 75–76
  workout program, 81–82
Water magic, 1–19
  choosing a pool, 12–13
  choosing your program, 4–8
  extra equipment, 13, 14–15
  muscles, 11–12, 16–17
  qualities of, 1–2
  safety tips, 18–19
  selecting a suit, 13
  setting your goals, 9–10
  testing the power of, 2–4
  waterpower is what you need, 4
Water parcourse, 134
Water tripping, 52
Wilkins, Mac, xv, 16, 126–27
Williams, Steve, 1
Workout schedule, 84–86
Wysocki, Ruth, xv, 136